SKILLS UPDATE

BOOK 4

Irene Heywood Jones
MSc, RGN, RMN, ONC, DipN, RNT
is a nurse tutor in orthopaedics and elderly care
at St Vincent's Hospital, Pinner,
and a freelance writer

ILLUSTRATED BY
Mike Bostock

EDITED BY
Sue Smith, RGN, RHV,
Professional Studies Editor
Nursing Times

DESIGNED BY
Hilary Tranter

FOREWORD

As increasing numbers of professional and informal
carers are involved in giving more care to people in the
community, there is a growing need for an understanding
of both simple and complex procedures affecting
patients and clients.

Skills Update 4,
the final collection of articles which first appeared in
Community Outlook, aims to update nurses on familiar
skills and give background information on new
procedures affecting their clients.

It is not intended to be a first-line teaching series for
acquiring new skills but, rather, to be used as an update
to encourage practitioners to reflect on skills
they may have learned some time ago or to provide an
overview of technical procedures experienced by
patients so that the best holistic care can be given,
whatever the environment.

The Skills Update books may prove useful as aids to
those who are teaching students and non-nurse carers
about treatments their clients or relatives are receiving.

Sue Smith
Professional Studies Editor, *Nursing Times*

CONTENTS

VENEPUNCTURE: US

WHO WILL PRESENT?

Any client who requiries blood sampling by venepuncture for:

- Estimation and measurement of blood components, for example, urea and electrolytes, lipids or hormones
- Part of pre-surgical preparation; for haemoglobin

estimation, full blood count and cross-matching prior to blood transfusion

- A post-surgical check of haemoglobin levels
- The detection of abnormalities, such as alphafetoprotein in pregnancy, glandular fever antibodies or rheumatoid factor.

SAFETY MEASURES

- Every client should be regarded as a potential biohazard.
- Latex or vinyl gloves must be worn when handling any blood products or bodily fluids.
- Protection of all personnel is paramount when handling blood products and bodily fluids. All staff must adhere to universal precautions and use appropriate barrier methods to prevent contamination.
- Needlestick injury is a potential source for many infections, but especially dangerous are the hepatitis B and HIV viruses transmitted in blood and bodily fluids.
- With a closed vacuum container system, such as the Vacutainer, a blood sample is transferred from the vein via a double-ended needle directly into the collecting tube which has a rubber stopper. The rear end of the needle has a retractable latex sleeve; this slides back to expose

the needle and allow penetration through the stopper of the collecting tube. Each time a tube is removed the protective sleeve automatically recovers and reseals the needle, so preventing blood seepage. This technique avoids the need for manual transfer from syringe to collecting tube, thereby minimising the handling of blood and the attendant dangers. It also ensures the biological integrity of the sample, as the exact amount required is drawn and blood comes into immediate contact with the additive.

- Always check that the tamperproof paper seal is intact to ensure sterility before using any needle to sample blood.
- Do not complete any information on the blood collection tubes until after the sample has been taken in order to avoid confusion with bottles and clients.

CHOOSING A SUITABLE VEIN

- Examine both arms to identify an accessible vein.
- Veins can be made more visible by applying a temporary tourniquet above the elbow and asking the client to hold the arm downwards and to clench the fist.
- Fine, thready or thrombosed veins are not suitable, nor are superficial 'floating' veins which tend to be mobile. Select a vein that is visible and fairly prominent or can be located by palpation. The usual choice is the basilic vein, the cephalic vein, the median cubital vein in the ante-cubital fossa or veins in the dorsal aspect of the hand.

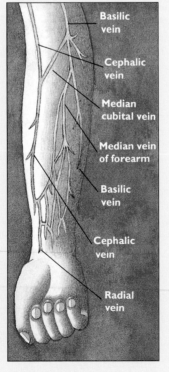

Basilic vein

Cephalic vein

Median cubital vein

Median vein of forearm

Basilic vein

Cephalic vein

Radial vein

DISPOSAL OF EQUIPMENT

- Keep gloves on while disposing of equipment, then dispose of gloves safely.
- Staff must be responsible for disposing of their own venepuncture equipment.
- Disposable needle holders are available. Alternatively, holders can be reused providing they are disinfected following current guidelines.
- If a needle disposal box is used, with needle on holder, place the needle hub into the tapered safety slot on top of the box. Move the hub along the taper until it is engaged securely. Untwist the needle, then slide holder back along the taper allowing the needle to drop into the box. On top of the box there is both a temporary and permanent lock.
- Another type of disposal container takes the complete needle and holder unit.
- An approved sharps container must not be filled beyond the designated capacity; it is then sealed and sent for incineration.
- Any other equipment which has been contaminated with blood should be disposed of appropriately or sterilised according to current policy.

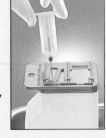

NG VACUUM TUBES

BLOOD SAMPLING TECHNIQUE

- You will need gloves, tray or receiver, tourniquet, appropriate collecting tubes with colour-coded stoppers to indicate type of preservative, manufacturer's guide, needle and a spare holder, skin cleansing swab, sterile wool or gauze swabs, skin plaster, pathology forms and pen.
- Explain the procedure to allay anxiety and ensure cooperation.
- Ensure the client is sitting or lying comfortably, with both arms free of clothing from the elbow down.
- Check the pathology request and appropriate collecting bottles.
- Identify a suitable vein for blood sampling and have the arm held downwards in extension on a secure surface.
- Wash and dry your hands and put on gloves.

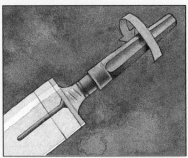

- Twist off the opaque shield to reveal the needle end covered by a latex sleeve. Screw this on to the holder, leaving the coloured sheath intact.
- Apply a tourniquet above the elbow and ask the client to clench his or her fist, which will raise the vein.
- Cleanse the skin area for 30 seconds and allow to dry. Unscrew the coloured sheath to reveal the needle and hold it with the bevel upwards.

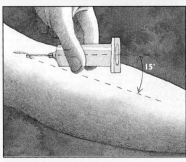

- Hold the skin taut over the vein. Using the holder like a syringe, insert the needle at an angle of 15° to enter the vein. Take care to remain in the lumen of the vein, rather than passing through the far side of the vessel.
- Once established in the vein, steady the holder with your non-dominant hand to anchor the needle in the

venepuncture site. With your dominant hand, place the collecting tube within the holder, grasp the holder wings between index and middle fingers and push the collecting tube in with the thumb until the rear needle pierces its stopper.

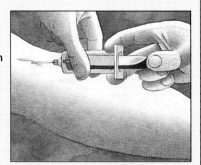

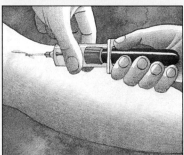

- A vacuum built into the collecting tube will extract precisely the predetermined amount required; the flow will stop automatically.
- Release the tourniquet when blood begins to flow.
- The tube is removed and gently rocked if the blood is to be mixed with an additive. Do not shake vigorously as this may cause haemolysis (breaking down of blood cells).
- By changing collecting tubes additional samples can be taken from the original venepuncture site. Order of collection is: tubes without additives; coagulation tubes; tubes with additives.
- Once completed, remove the needle from the client's arm/hand while pressing a sterile wool or gauze swab on to the venepuncture site to stem the leakage of blood.
- Ask the client to press on the site, applying digital pressure for at least one minute, and flex the elbow, which also raises the arm. Check that the client feels well.
- Dispose of all equipment safely in approved containers.
- Check that the wound site has stopped bleeding and apply a skin plaster if required. Only then dispose of gloves and wash hands.
- Check pathology forms against client's details and complete these on the collecting tubes.

NOW YOU SHOULD FEEL COMPETENT TO:

- Understand how to obtain blood samples from a venepuncture site using the vacuum container system.

FURTHER READING
Thorpe, S. *A Practical Guide to Taking Blood.* London: Baillière Tindall, 1991. Royal College of Nursing. *Universal Precautions.* London: RCN, 1993.

Note: It is advisable that nurses new to the technique undergo a period of supervised practice with an experienced phlebotomy practitioner to ensure competency. The Skills Update series is intended to encourage nurses to reflect on and update their practice. It is not intended to teach new skills.

EYE CARE

WHO MAY PRESENT

Clients requiring eye medications and mydriatics to dilate the pupils before eye examinations. In particular:

- Those requiring topical antibiotics, either as prophylaxis after surgery or to treat infections such as those causing conjunctivitis and blepharitis; also agents to treat herpes
- Those requiring the instillation of topical anti-allergy and anti-inflammatory agents, such as steroids
- Those needing artificial tears for dry eyes, often associated with rheumatoid conditions, exophthalmos and facial paralysis.
- Miotic drugs to constrict the pupils in cases of glaucoma.

POINTS TO REMEMBER

- Great care is necessary to prevent cross-infection, especially from one eye to the other.
- Ensure that medications are being stored correctly, as some require refrigeration, and check they are still within the date for use.
- Eye preparations should never be shared between clients.
- Always sweep from the inner canthus (nasal side) to the outer canthus to minimise risk of cross-infection.
- Ensure medication applicators touch no part of the eye, both to prevent contamination of the preparation and prevent damage to the eye.

GENERAL PREPARATION

- Ensure that the operator has a good light source but that the client is not dazzled.
- Explain the procedure to the client and elicit his or her cooperation. Make sure you know which eye is to be treated. Ensure the client is seated or reclining comfortably with the head supported and neck slightly extended.
- It is often easier to work from behind the client and may provide less distraction. The operator's dominant hand can rest on the client's forehead, giving an extra margin of safety; should the person move inadvertently the hand will move with him or her.
- By asking the client to look upwards, this effectively moves the cornea away from the possible danger of accidental damage.
- Provide the client with a tissue to dab excess fluids.
- Before administering medications, remove any discharge or crusts by wiping gently along the lid margins from within outwards, using a cotton-wool ball moistened with cooled boiled water. Do not use dry wool balls as fibres may get into the eye.

- If several different preparations are to be administered to the same eye, leave a few minutes' interval between medications to avoid a dilution effect. With combined prescriptions for drops and ointment, put drops in first as the greasy ointment can inhibit absorption of drops.
- Be alert for any systemic reactions, such as bronchospasm or bradycardia, associated with drugs absorbed into the circulation.
- Advise clients that their vision may be impaired while receiving eye preparations and encourage them to take special care. After mydriatics such as tropicamide 5%, used to dilate the pupil and facilitate examination, there will be difficulty in focusing and clients must not drive until normal vision is completely restored.
- If the medication is being administered after surgery, check other instructions the client was given on discharge: such as not bending the head forwards; use of eye pads, shields or dark glasses; washing hair backwards over a basin; not lifting heavy objects; advice on participating in sports.

APPLICATION OF OINTMENTS

- Prepare the client, check that the preparation is the correct one and remove the screw cap of the tube.
- Pull gently on skin below the eye to evert the lower lid and ask client to look upwards.
- Squeeze the tube and form a ribbon of ointment 2cm long.
- Hold the tube clear of the eye while applying the ribbon just inside the lid margin at the inner canthus, moving along to the outer side, squeezing out the ointment as required.
- If applied correctly the procedure should not cause the client to blink.
- Encourage the client to open and close the eye twice in order to get the ointment on both lids.

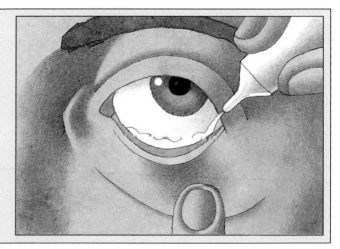

INSTILLING EYE DROPS

- Check the dropper bottle, prepare the patient and have tissues at hand.
- Unscrew the dropper bottle or, for those with a separate pipette, squeeze bulb to fill the dropper.
- Rest two fingers on the skin below the eye and gently draw down to expose the lower fornix, comprising the conjunctival sac.
- Ask client to look upwards and empty contents of dropper with one firm squeeze into the sac nearer the outer canthus, as this will limit loss down the nasolacrimal passage.
- Ensure the client keeps head tilted back while blinking gently, without squeezing the eyelids, to retain as much fluid as possible.
- Excess fluid from cheeks should then be dabbed, but do not rub the eyeball.

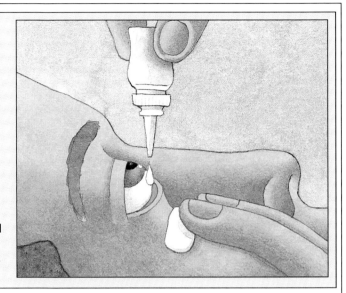

SELF-ADMINISTRATION OF EYE DROPS

- Prescriptions may require eye drops to be administered at frequent intervals and over a long period, so it is obviously easier and more cost-effective if the client or carer can be taught to do this.
- An automatic dropper is a cheap and simple way of improving self-administration of eye drops that are in plastic containers. The dropper bottle slots into a collar and is secured by a clip-on portion ensuring that it is correctly positioned over the eye. The client holds down the lower eyelid and fixes the appliance around the eye, ensuring the small lip is against the cheek; this prevents blinking. The client then tilts the head back and, by looking through a small pinhole, his or her view is aimed upwards. One squeeze and the bottle delivers the eye drops accurately and safely. Between treatments the plastic dropper appliance should be washed under hot water or may be boiled, as indicated in the manufacturers' instructions. It is discarded after treatment is concluded.
- Another automatic device makes grasping and squeezing a dropper bottle more manageable for clients who have a weak grip or difficulty with fine finger movements. This is a plastic device that fits securely around the dropper bottle and provides a wider handling base. It may be used in conjunction with the dropper applicator.

1. Place the keyhole slot around the base of the bottle neck below the thread and close the automatic dropper device.

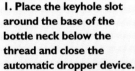

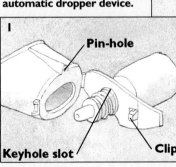

2. Hold down the lower eyelid and place the device over the eye with the lip against the cheek

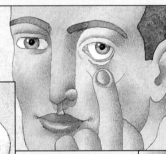

3. Tilt the head backwards and look through the pin-hole towards the light

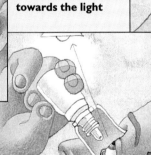

4. Squeeze the bottle gently to allow the drops to fall into the eye

NOW YOU SHOULD FEEL COMPETENT TO:

- Apply ointment and instil drops into clients' eyes as required
- Instruct and support clients and their carers in the self-administration of eye drops and ointments.

FURTHER READING

Stollery, R. *Ophthalmic Nursing*. Oxford: Blackwell Scientific Publications, 1987.

RING P

WHO MAY PRESENT?

Women who require a change of ring pessary in order to correct a uterine prolapse— predominately older post-menopausal women. It is the treatment of choice when clients:

- Are unfit for major surgery to repair the condition
- Decide not to undergo surgery
- Prefer a palliative treatment to control symptoms
- Need a temporary measure while awaiting surgery.

UTERINE PROLAPSE

- Prolapse is the downward displacement or herniation of the uterus and/or vaginal walls. It occurs when there is laxity and weakening of the supporting ligaments and pelvic floor muscles.
- It may be associated with obstetric trauma and poor postnatal exercising. Ninety-nine per cent of prolapses occur in women who have borne children; it is rarely found in nulliparous women.
- Prolapse often becomes evident following the menopause when there is atrophy of the pelvic ligaments through loss of oestrogen, together with diminished muscle tone.
- It is aggravated by raised intra-abdominal pressure, as with coughing, sneezing, laughing, straining on defecation and lifting heavy objects. This may include carers moving dependants.
- There are three stages of prolapse:
— First degree. The uterus descends, but the cervix remains within the vagina.
— Second degree. The cervix protrudes from the vaginal orifice.
— Third degree. The uterus lies outside the vagina.
- Client may complain of:
— Feeling of 'something coming down' or 'falling out'
— Presence of a lump or protrusion at the vulva
— Offensive blood-stained discharge from tissue friction
— Pressure in pelvis or a dragging sensation
— Difficulty in walking or sitting comfortably
— Urinary symptoms of dysuria, frequency, infection or stress incontinence
— Symptoms worse at the end of the day or after prolonged standing or straining
— Social and sexual embarrassment and limitation of activities.

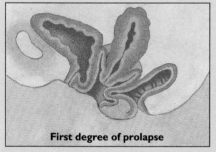

First degree of prolapse

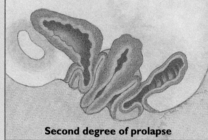

Second degree of prolapse

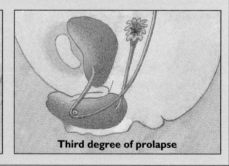

Third degree of prolapse

SELECTION OF PESSARY

- Ring pessaries come in a size range of 50–110mm in diameter. Those most commonly used are between 68mm and 79mm. They are supplied in sterile packaging for single use.
- A ring pessary is compressible by hand but springs back to its circular shape once inside the vagina. The polythene type is fairly rigid but can be made more pliable by immersion in hot water prior to use. The PVC vinyl type is made of a naturally flexible material.
- The positioning of a ring pessary effectively supports in a sling fashion, keeping the vaginal walls taut and holding up the uterus.
- The first ring pessary will be inserted by a gynaecologist or GP who will conduct a thorough examination and select the appropriate size: one that can be rotated while in the vagina
by the doctor and will remain in place even when the woman is straining.
- Once inserted into the vagina, the woman should not feel any discomfort or even be aware of the presence of the ring pessary. If too large, it will give rise to internal discomfort and may cause pressure necrosis and ulceration.
- When established in place, the ring pessary will need to be changed every three to six months, depending on the clinical protocol. This provides an opportunity to examine the vagina and cervix and evaluate their condition.

SSARIES

INSERTION OF PESSARY

- The woman should be given an explanation of the procedure and its aims and shown the ring pessary.
- She should pass urine and swab the vulval area from front to back with clean water.
- The woman should be asked to remove pants, corsets, stockings or tights and to lie on the couch covered by a modesty sheet.
- The nurse should wash her hands and put on latex gloves.
- The size of the ring pessary should be checked against the prescription and removed from its sealed sterile packaging.
- If the nurse immerses the pessary in a bowl of hot water to make it more pliable, she must be extremely careful that it has cooled before putting it into the client's vagina.
- The woman should be asked to lie on her back, with her knees drawn up and separated. Alternatively the practitioner may prefer to use the left lateral position.
- The nurse should use a vaginal speculum to examine for any areas of excoriation, irritation, ulceration or discharge. If any abnormalities are detected, these should be referred to the GP before a new pessary is inserted.
- With the thumb and forefinger of the dominant hand, the pessary should be compressed into an oval shape, then a water-based lubricant should be applied.
- Using the non-dominant hand, the nurse should part the labia to expose the entrance to the vagina.
- The nurse should slide the pessary into the posterior part of the vagina, pushing backwards and downwards until it settles in the posterior fornix. The pessary will spring back to its circular shape once inside the vagina above the pelvic floor.

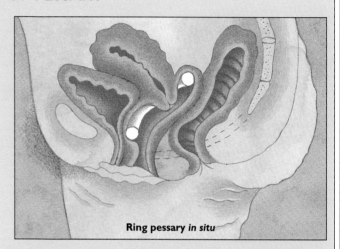

Ring pessary *in situ*

- When secured posteriorly, the nurse should hook the front portion of the pessary into the anterior fornix of the vagina, secured behind the symphysis pubis. The cervix will be seen positioned centrally through the ring.
- The client should be asked whether the pessary feels comfortable. She should sit up, stand up and walk around, cough, bear down and ideally have a bowel movement to ensure the fit is secure.
- The nurse should check that the client understands about the management of the ring pessary and that she has instructions for her observations.
- An appointment should be made for a future check and change and a name and telephone number should be given to the client for her to contact if any problems occur.

INFORMATION FOR THE CLIENT

- Once *in situ*, the woman should be unaware of the presence of the ring pessary. If there is any discomfort, this may indicate that a different size is needed or that there is a localised problem in the vagina.
- When a ring pessary is used for older women past the menopause, they may experience dryness as a result of atrophic vaginitis and be prone to abrading, irritation and ulceration. Oestrogen cream may be prescribed for topical application to the vagina to improve the quality of the tissue and can be used in conjunction with a ring pessary.

- It is quite common for women with a ring pessary to experience a slight watery discharge. This can be managed effectively by using pant liners.
- The woman should seek prompt medical attention for any discharge that is purulent, frothy, curd-like, offensive, irritating or blood-stained.
- A ring pessary should not interfere with micturition or bowel action, and sexual intercourse is possible.
- The client should be advised to continue normal vulval cleansing daily, using bath, shower or bidet.

NOW YOU SHOULD FEEL COMPETENT TO:

- Change a ring pessary, after supervised practice
- Advise clients on the use of ring pessaries and the necessary observations.

BREAST AND TESTICUL

- Women or men attending a clinic or surgery who express concern about cancer owing to a personal or family history of the condition or who mention it as a result of heightened awareness of breast or testicular cancer
- Clients attending well-women or well-men clinics
- New patients registering at a general practice.

BREAST SELF-EXAMINATION TECHNIQUE

- Breast examination should be undertaken after menstruation, as pre-menstrually there is uncharacteristic swelling and lumpiness of the breast. It can also be tender and painful to handle. This timing serves as a regular reminder to be 'breast aware'.
- The patient should be encouraged to identify what is normal for her and be familiar with the areas of the breast and axilla. Most women can expect one breast to be larger than the other.
- She should stand with her hands by her side in front of the mirror and look at the breasts from the front and while rotating the upper body from side to side.
- With the palms of hands resting on the hips she should press down firmly and pull back the shoulders. This will cause flexing of the chest muscles and allow for checking of the breasts from side to side.
- With hands on her head, she should look carefully for any dimples, swelling or 'orange peel' appearance on the breast or in the axilla.
- Placing the hands over the head will enable the patient to look carefully under the breasts and at the nipple areas.
- Next she should lie down with a pillow or folded towel under her non-dominant shoulder and that arm raised and held behind the head. It is easier to do the initial palpation with the dominant hand.
- Using the flat surface of the fingers, she should press gently on the breast tissue, moving around in a circle, as if following a clock face. She should start at the 12 o'clock position at the upper part of the breast, commencing at the nipple and working back round to the start. She should move out by two finger-breadths and repeat this circular motion, radiating out until the whole breast has been examined.
- Finally she should feel up into the tail of the breast and axilla. Then she should gently pinch the nipple between thumb and finger to ensure there is no secretion.
- She should repeat this sequence on the other breast.
- The client may find the procedure more comfortable and easier to do while in the bath, using a wet, soapy hand that slides over the breasts.
- Abnormalities will manifest as:
  — Alteration in shape of the breast
  — Nipple changing direction, turning inwards or at an unusual angle
  — Lumps on or within the breast tissue or axilla
  — Thickened areas of tissue or a hard knot
  — Bulging or swelling on the breast surface or axilla
  — 'Orange peel' skin, as if there is an area of tethering under the surface
  — Dimples or puckering
  — Areola swelling or puckering
  — Discharge from the nipple, either serous or blood.
- Mastitis will manifest as tenderness and a feeling of heaviness in the breast; there may be a discharge of pus from the nipple as a result of bacterial infection.

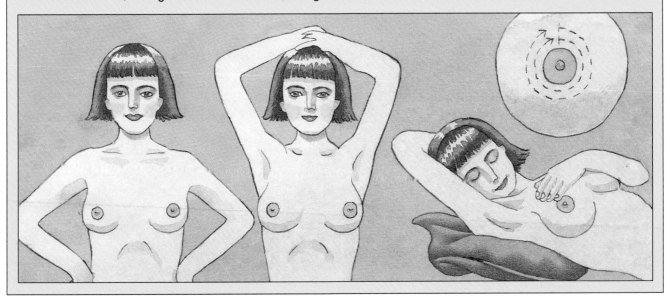

R SELF-EXAMINATION

TESTICULAR SELF-EXAMINATION TECHNIQUE

- Examination should take place in or after a bath or shower when the scrotal sac is warm and relaxed, with the testes hanging loose.
- The patient should understand the normal composition of the scrotum, the testes and the epididymis.
- He should be taught to cup the scrotum and support it in the palm of the hand to note the size and weight of the testes. One testicle can be expected to hang below the other and one will feel slightly larger.
- He should gently palpate each testicle. Using both hands, the testicle should be rolled between the thumb and forefingers.
- The testicle should feel egg-shaped, smooth on the surface and firm. The epididymis, along the top and behind the testicle, will have the texture of soft rope or cord. If the scrotum is warm and relaxed the epididymis will easily separate from the testicle.
- If an irregularity is suspected, the other testicle will serve as a comparison.
- Abnormalities will manifest as:
  — An increase in the size or weight of the testes or a heaviness in the scrotum
  — Lumps or swellings
  — A non-smooth, irregular surface
  — Alteration in the firmness of the testes
  — A dull ache in the lower abdomen or groin
  — Possible swelling of the male breasts (gynaecomastia).
- This cancer occurs most commonly in younger men and is readily amenable to a cure if treated early.
- Other conditions that manifest as changes in appearance and feel of the scrotal sac include hydrocele, orchitis and epididymitis.

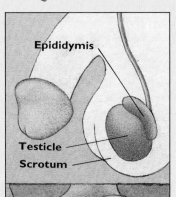

Epididymis

Testicle

Scrotum

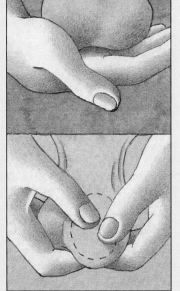

GENERAL ADVICE

- Clients should be taught constant self-awareness, rather than obsessive self-examination.
- Encourage clients to be familiar with the natural feel and contours of their bodies so they are alert to changes.
- It is helpful to explain and demonstrate the examination procedure, point out normally occurring lumpiness in breast tissue and the epididymis in the testes. A professional examination will establish and confirm a normality baseline. A model breast is a useful aid.
- Nurses must be aware that clients may be embarrassed to perform and to be observed performing these self-examination techniques.
- Abnormalities are often detected by sexual partners.
- Breast cancer is not unknown in men.
- Testicular self-examination should, ideally, be introduced into school health education.

ALTERATIONS FROM NORMAL

- Clients detecting any change from their norm must be advised to seek medical advice as soon as possible, but remember that fear of cancer is still prevalent. Try to dispel this fear. Most changes will not be caused by cancer, but this needs to be excluded. In fact nine out of 10 breast lumps prove to be benign.
- It is crucial to emphasise that early detection and prompt treatment offers the greatest chance of successful cure for any type of cancer. While continuing to reassure, advise clients not to wait to see whether the symptoms disappear but to get them checked out.

NOW YOU SHOULD FEEL COMPETENT TO:

- Advise clients on how to perform breast or testicular self-examination.

RESOURCES
McCormack Ltd, Church House, Church Square, Leighton Buzzard, Bedfordshire LU7 7AE. Tel: 01525 851313.
Northamptonshire Health Promotion, Beaumont Villa, Cliftonville, Northampton NN1 5BE. Tel: 01604 35681.
Yorkshire Regional Cancer Organisation, Cookridge Hospital, Leeds LS16 6QB. Tel: 01132 673411.
All the above provide leaflets on testicular self-examination.
Imperial Cancer Research Fund, PO Box 123, Lincoln's Inn Fields, London WC2A 3PX. Tel: 0171-242 0200. Provides leaflets on breast self-examination.

STOMA CARE

WHO MAY PRESENT?

- Any client who has a colostomy, ileostomy or urostomy
— Most clients will have had access to a stoma care nurse following surgery. For those having elective surgery, the stoma care nurse would ideally be involved pre-operatively
— The stoma care nurse would aim to do a follow-up visit at home and later on in the stoma clinic. The district nurse will also be asked about stoma care and may liaise with the specialist stoma nurse
- Silent ostomates: clients who have had a stoma fashioned many years ago may seek assistance as they get older, as their faculties or manual dexterity diminish or other circumstances change.

BACKGROUND INFORMATION

- An ileostomy is formed if the whole of the colon is removed, for example, in ulcerative colitis. In Crohn's disease the colon may sometimes be rested by the formation of an ileostomy. These clients tend to be under 45 when the operation is performed.
— The ileum end is drawn out of the abdominal wall, everted and sutured to the skin. The stoma is shaped like a spout and the output is of liquid or 'porridge' consistency.
- A colostomy is an opening into the colon, bringing the large bowel to the surface of the abdominal wall, for example, after surgery for bowel cancer, intractable faecal incontinence, diverticulitis or paraplegia/spinal dysfunction. The solidity of the faeces depends upon the colostomy site, with a more formed stool found nearer the descending colon and rectum.

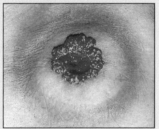

A typical 'rosebud' shape colostomy

— A permanent colostomy is flush with the skin surface and like a rosebud shape. Clients may also be coping with the effects of the associated surgery; these clients tend to be above 50 and often considerably older.
- A urostomy is fashioned to enable urine to be excreted via an abdominal stoma, in cases of spinal dysfunction or excision of the bladder, often for cancer.

STOMA APPLIANCES

- A urostomy bag has a tap mechanism with a tactile spot to indicate if the tap is open or closed.
- A stoma bag of the drainable type is used for an ileostomy, or a colostomy in the ascending colon, which collects effluent of a porridge-like consistency. One bag is used for about 24 hours and has a drainable end that is held secure with ties or a clip. It is important that these are affixed properly to ensure safe closure and no leakage.
- A colostomy bag to collect solid faeces is a closed bag.
- A one-piece bag has a sticky flange that is applied directly to the skin.
- A two-piece system has a separate flange that is applied to the skin and can remain in place for about three to five days. Bags are attached by a clip-on seal.
- Bags are available in a cosmetic opaque, flesh colour, or clear for the poorly sighted or those who need to visualise their stoma when applying the bag.
- The whole of the flange must be a precise fit over the stoma to avoid leakage and sore skin. About three to four weeks post-surgery the stoma will normally have settled to its regular size. Clients may need to cut the flange opening to fit the stoma size and shape.
- The choice of stoma appliance is made on advice from the specialist nurse, who considers the stoma site, client preference, lifestyle and ability. The two-piece system and the drainable bag clip closures can be difficult for clients with poor eyesight, tremor or manual dexterity problems, to manipulate.

LIFESTYLE ISSUES

- Body image — there needs to be a period of bereavement and adjustment to the altered body image for client, partner and close family members. Counselling and help from relevant self-help groups and other adjusted ostomates can be very beneficial.[1]
- Clothing — ideally the stoma is sited away from the waistband so that normal clothing can be worn. For elderly clients who have lax abdominal muscles, it is possible to have a special support girdle, available on prescription, made to accommodate the stoma bag.
- Odour — with a well-fitting flange and a regular change of bag, odour should present no greater a problem than normal bowel function; many bags contain an integral odour filter.
- Diet — ostomates can eat as normal, although they may be advised to be aware of foods such as baked beans, peppers, cabbage and onions which tend to produce flatus.
- Activities — clients may wish to discuss how best to resume activities such as swimming, tennis, dancing and sex. There are various devices for use in these situations, which stoma care nurses can advise on.

STOMA MANAGEMENT

■ The client or nurse should collect the necessary equipment:
— Prepared bag and flange
— Accessories, for example, spare clips, filler or powder if required
— Scissors
— Bowl of warm water, or ascertain easy access to sink
— Skin wipes such as flannels or gauze swabs but not cotton wool or tissues as these disintegrate and stick to the skin
— Clean latex gloves for the nurse or carer
— Disposal bags and newspaper or nappy sacks.

■ The client should select a suitable place and time to attend to stoma care — in the bathroom or on the commode.

■ Remove the bag or flange gently, supporting the surrounding skin. Wipe around the flange site and actual stoma and wash with warm water and mild unperfumed soap if necessary.

■ Check the state of the peristomal skin:
— A change of adhesive appliance may be needed if there is an allergic reaction or irritation
— Soreness or irritation may be due to a poor fit between the flange and stoma permitting leakage; this may indicate that reassessment of the flange hole size is necessary. If there are bumps and indentations of the skin around the

stoma, which are impeding close fitting of the appliance, the client is shown how to smooth out the surface by using a filler or a malleable cohesive flange

— If soreness persists apply a stoma cream or a stoma powder if the skin is weeping; apply sparingly to the affected area before applying flange.

■ Observe stoma for prolapse, retraction, necrosis or peristomal hernia.

■ Ensure the peristomal skin is perfectly dry, then attach a new flange or bag, ensuring these are close fitting to the stoma and secured safely.

■ Disposal of stoma equipment:
— When emptying a drainable bag, the client should lean over the toilet or commode, or sit well back on the seat and part legs. Remove the clip attachment and allow waste matter to pass into the toilet, wipe the end of the bag then reattach clip.
— When removing a closed bag, hold it over the toilet, cut the end and expel faecal waste into the toilet. As the toilet flushes, hold the bag under the water flow and allow it to pass through the top of the bag and out at the bottom to flush through. The same procedure is repeated when finally disposing of a drainable bag. Put into a disposal bag and seal.
— Stoma appliances can be disposed of in household waste.

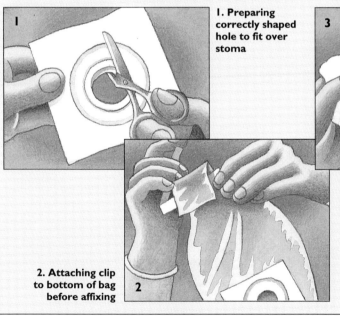

1. Preparing correctly shaped hole to fit over stoma

2. Attaching clip to bottom of bag before affixing

3. Preparing to fix bag over ileostomy site

4. Fixing bag on to skin around stoma

RESOURCES

■ British Colostomy Association,
15 Station Road,
Reading,
Berkshire RG1 1LG
Tel: 01734 391537

■ Ileostomy Association
Amblehurst House,
PO Box 23, Mansfield,

Nottinghamshire
NG18 4TT.
Tel: 01623 28099.

■ Urostomy Association
Buckland,
Beaumont Park,
Danbury,
Essex CM3 4DE
Tel: 01245 224294

NOW YOU SHOULD BE AWARE OF:

■ The needs of clients with a stoma.
■ Where to seek further information on living with a stoma.

REFERENCE
1. Price, B., Smith, S. Stoma and body image. *Community Outlook* 1991; 1: 8, 21–24.

ADMINISTRATIO

WHO MAY PRESENT?

- Clients requiring an evacuant enema for the relief of constipation
- Clients needing bowel preparation for investigations such as abdominal X-ray, barium enema, proctoscopy or sigmoidoscopy or before surgery or childbirth
- A client who needs regular administration of retention enemas as topical treatment for bowel disorders such as ulcerative colitis.

WHAT YOU WILL NEED

- Enema preparation as prescribed
- Lubricating gel
- Bowl with warm water
- Plastic sheet and disposable drape
- Gamgee pad or toilet tissue
- Disposable gloves
- Disposal bag
- Bedpan or commode
- Good light source

ENEMA PREPARATIONS AND THEIR ACTIONS

- **Microenema**
  These are useful for moderate constipation or bowel preparation and are safe for adults and children over three years. Because of the low volume, a mere 5ml, it minimises discomfort and is easy to administer. They act by attracting water to bulk out the stool and stimulate defecation and also contain an agent to soften and lubricate the stool. Response usually occurs within five to 15 minutes.
- **Phosphate enema**
  The phosphate solution is hypertonic and water diffuses into the colon, causing the faeces to swell which in turn stimulates the defecatory reflex. Patients should be encouraged to drink plenty of water when on a course of phosphate enemas.
- **Arachis oil retention enema**
  This is indicated for impacted faeces and has the dual action of softening the faeces and lubricating the bowel. After administration clients should remain lying for as long as possible to ensure retention and enhance the action, ideally for at least 15–30 minutes.
- **Medicated retention enema**
  Two types are in use, mesalazine and prednisolone, both for the local treatment of ulcerative colitis. These are usually administered once daily, preferably at bedtime, to facilitate retention and allow the medication to work effectively. The container must be shaken well before use.

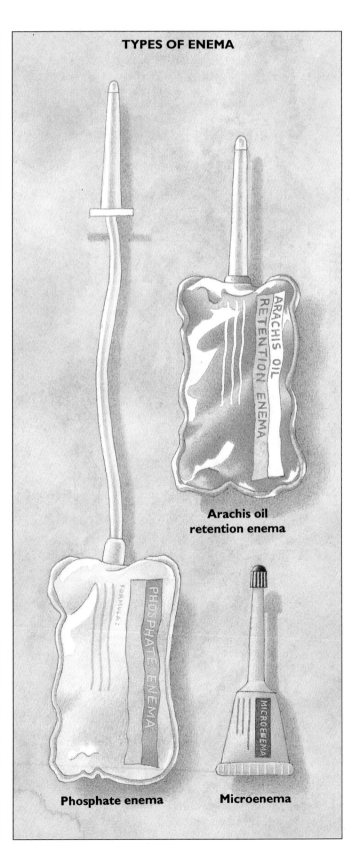

TYPES OF ENEMA

Arachis oil retention enema

Phosphate enema

Microenema

N OF ENEMAS

ENEMA ADMINISTRATION TECHNIQUE

- Ensure privacy and explain what you are about to do and why, to gain the client's consent and cooperation, especially regarding timing for retention of the enema.
- Ask client to remove lower garments, but ensure modesty and warmth by covering with a sheet or blanket.
- Ask client to lie in left lateral position with knees flexed, upper one higher than lower, and buttocks close to the edge of the bed. This accords with the anatomical position of the colon, and gravity will help the passage of fluid.
- Added comfort can be gained by placing the head on one pillow and the top arm holding another pillow close to the chest.
- Protect the bed with a plastic sheet and disposable drape tucked under the buttocks.
- Reassure the client that a bedpan or commode is at hand or ensure that the lavatory will be available.
- Place disposable enema pack in bowl of water warm to the touch (not necessary with microenemas).
- Sit beside the client with a good light source aimed at the anal area. Put on disposable gloves as protection against intestinal-borne micro-organisms, especially hepatitis A.
- Make an initial examination of the perianal area, checking for soreness, inflammation, fissures, skin tags or haemorrhoids, anal distension, rectal prolapse or bleeding. If indicated, also perform a digital examination of the bowel using a lubricated finger, noting the extent of constipation or impaction. Then change gloves.
- Warn client that the enema is about to be administered and that he or she will feel a tube entering the anus. The person should be advised to take deep breaths. This provides a means of distraction and encourages relaxation.
- Remove the plastic tip from the nozzle of the disposable enema. Lubricate the nozzle if required, although some manufacturers say a drop of the fluid content is sufficient lubricant.
- Ensure all air is expelled from the nozzle. Part the buttocks and pass the full length of the pliable nozzle gently into the anal canal without exerting force.
- Expel all the fluid from the pack slowly and gently by squeezing and rolling the pack to prevent backflow. Remove the nozzle, with container still compressed, and dispose of the enema pack.
- Wipe the anal area and put a pad or tissues to the anus as protection from leakage. Leave the client comfortable with a reminder of how long to retain the preparation.
- After the client has had a bowel action, observe the stools and report on the contents, quantity and consistency.
- Check before leaving that the patient feels comfortable, has no abdominal pain, cramps, distention or flatus.
- This procedure may need to be taught to a carer. Alternatively a client may be able to perform an enema on himself or herself and there are tube extensions for this purpose which may be advanced 6–8cm into the rectum.

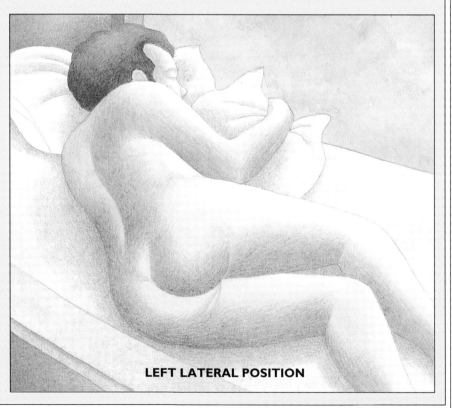

LEFT LATERAL POSITION

NOW YOU SHOULD BE AWARE OF:

- The needs of patients requiring enemas at home and how to administer various types of enema.

PRE-SURGERY

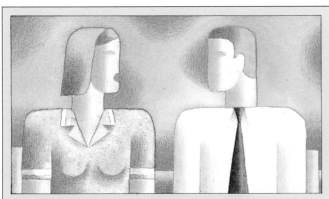

WHO MAY PRESENT?

■ Clients who are undergoing elective surgical procedures, such as gynaecological, ophthalmological, orthopaedic, abdominal or bowel operations. Also clients having day surgery and requiring certain complex investigations, such as endoscopy or myelogram.

■ Clients attending a health centre to have a pre-surgery checklist completed, including tests and examinations. This may be requested when there is a cross-boundary referral to a distant hospital. They may need to attend a hospital for investigations such as X-ray or ECG.

■ Clients requiring specific information about an operation or help and advice on pre-surgery preparation, such as instilling eye drops or creams, vaginal preparations, enemas or suppositories.

■ Clients attending a surgeon's outreach clinic in a health centre where group bookings for surgery are planned.

Clients may attend a hospital pre-assessment clinic or be visited by nurse specialists at home.

AIMS OF PRE-SURGERY PREPARATION

■ To ensure the client is fully prepared and in optimum health in order to provide the best circumstances for safe and uncomplicated surgery and recovery.

■ To identify any problems or at-risk factors that may undermine the surgery or anaesthesia.

■ To minimise the risks of post-operative complications by treating existing medical conditions before surgery.

■ To eliminate unnecessary admission to hospital where the client is found to be unfit for surgery. This is wasteful of operating time and distressing for the client and family.

■ To provide an opportunity for health education regarding peri-operative risks associated with smoking, alcohol consumption, exercise, diet and excess weight; also to acquaint the client with his or her role in the rehabilitation process.

■ To provide an opportunity for the client's anxieties to be voiced and be dealt with at the same time or referred to the appropriate professional.

■ For the client who has not had a routine health check, this surgical event may be the first opportunity for a health assessment and any hidden problems to be identified.

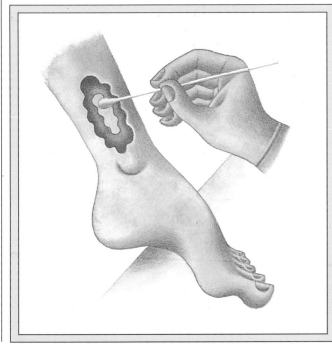

PHYSICAL SCREENING

The following procedures may be undertaken:

■ Urine testing — screening for urinary tract infection, kidney dysfunction or diabetes mellitus

■ Blood tests — full blood count, urea and electrolytes and haemoglobin; screening for anaemia and electrolyte imbalance

■ ECG and chest X-ray — requested if indicated and may be routine protocol for clients over a certain age, variously from 45 to 60

■ Swabs — to ensure the operation site is free from infection

■ Respiration — noting any breathlessness or cough as well as smoking habits

■ Blood pressure — screening for hypertension

■ Temperature and pulse — to give baseline values and to screen for infection

■ Weight and height — screen for malnourishment, obesity and dehydration; also provide a guide for the anaesthetist.

PREPARATION

OBSERVATIONS AND INFORMATION TO NOTE

- Skin condition — general condition, allergy, rash, weeping or irritation, open wounds or sores
- Infection — respiratory tract, mouth sores, infected nail, conjunctivitis, urinary tract or vaginal infection, dental caries
- Circulation — colour, cyanosis, palor, capillary refill, oedema, varicose veins or leg ulcer
- Medical history — any details relevant to forthcoming surgery
- Current medications — particularly relevant are anticoagulants, antibiotics, hypotensives, steroids, hormone replacement therapy and the contraceptive pill
- Nursing history — difficulties that could affect the client's surgery, recovery and rehabilitation; for example, communication, sensory or mobility problems, dietary restrictions or specific dietary requirements, sleep, incontinence, constipation, domestic circumstances.

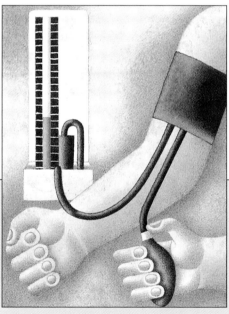

Opposite page, bottom left: taking swabs; right: urinalysis. This page, left: taking blood pressure; Below: taking blood

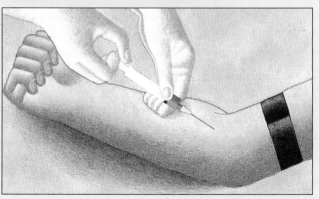

CLIENT/FAMILY EDUCATION

A well-prepared, well-informed client experiences less anxiety and less pain, makes a speedier recovery and is subject to fewer post-operative complications. The nurse should address individual concerns and identify information gaps in areas such as:

- Understanding the impending operation process and its objectives
- Pre-operative events regarding tests and preparation routine. Often clients are instructed to go into hospital on the morning of the operation day without breakfast, following a bath and perhaps after some type of bowel preparation
- Immediate post-operative recovery phase, so that clients are prepared for intravenous infusion or blood transfusion, wound drainage, oxygen, catheter or nasogastric tube, positioning, patient-controlled anaesthesia, leg and chest exercises
- The client's role in the rehabilitation programme and the role of physiotherapy, occupational therapy, as well as specialist nurse input, prostheses and aids to daily living
- Discharge planning arrangements and a recovery timetable for activities such as resuming work, sport, driving and sexual relations. Reassurance that there will be support from health centre staff and community nurses on return home, for this is often a time when clients feel most isolated and vulnerable
- Questions that cannot be answered — clients can be advised to write these down and to ask hospital staff on admission for surgery.

Patient information leaflets are available on many routine elective operations, with helpful diagrams and clear explanations, addressing common questions asked by patients.

Nurses in the community should become familiar with the protocols of local surgical teams in order to inform clients as fully as possible prior to admission.

NOW YOU SHOULD BE AWARE OF THE NEED TO:

- Undertake pre-surgery assessment requirements
- Offer advice and information to prepare clients before surgery or to direct them to the appropriate health care professional.

VAGINAL C

WHO MAY PRESENT?

■ Women who are experiencing vulval irritation or soreness, vaginal discharge, malodour, painful intercourse, urethritis or vaginal dryness

■ Women with confirmed vaginal infections or other conditions who require assistance with topical vaginal medication and advice to prevent recurrence.

■ Those attending a well woman clinic where discussion can include advice on maintaining vaginal health.

APPLICATION OF VAGINAL PREPARATIONS

■ Vaginal medication is available in the form of pessaries, creams and tablets:

— A pessary is medication packed into a solid cone shape which melts on contact with the vaginal walls

— Cream is inserted by filling an applicator with a measured dose and depositing it by use of a plunger (pre-filled applicators are also available)

— A vaginal tablet is similar to a pessary and should be inserted with an applicator.

■ Prepare the woman by explaining the importance of the procedure and how it is to be conducted. Demonstrate the pessary, tablet or cream applicator and describe how these must be placed high into the posterior fornix of the vagina. Clients might prefer instructions on self-administration. Others may require assistance from a nurse or carer.

■ Ensure the bed has a protective covering and that the client has a modesty sheet over the abdomen.

■ Ideally, medications should be administered before bedtime when the client is recumbent and will not lose medication from the orifice. After washing her hands, she should take the cream applicator and ensure the plunger is fully pushed in. The cream should be squeezed from the tube into the applicator (see diagram). Remove the tube. A vaginal tablet or pessary may be inserted into its applicator.

■ The client should lie on the bed with knees up. She should part the labia, locate the introitus and insert the applicator into the vagina. It should go in as far as is comfortable, about 8–10cm, aiming up and backwards. Once in place, the plunger is pushed in until it stops in order to deliver the tablet or dose of cream. The applicator should be thoroughly cleansed or disposed of safely. To insert a pessary, the procedure is similar, ensuring that the pessary is placed high in the vagina.

■ If the nurse assists with these procedures she must wear disposable gloves.

■ The client may be advised to wear a protective pad or panty liner to absorb any leakage.

■ These medications can be administered during menstruation. Intercourse is best avoided until the infection has cleared up.

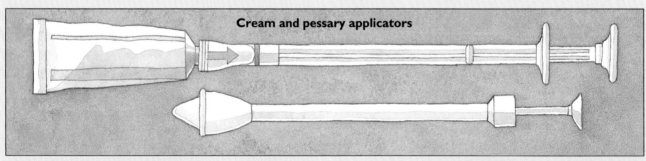

Cream and pessary applicators

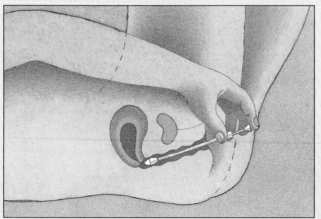
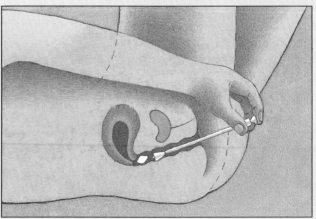

ONDITIONS

ADVICE FOR WOMEN ON MAINTAINING VAGINAL HEALTH

■ It is important to sustain the correct pH balance and temperature for a healthy vagina. Wear cotton underwear rather than nylon and change it regularly. To allow free air circulation around the perineum, avoid thick tights and close-fitting trousers.

■ Douche only on medical advice; otherwise do not apply commercial sprays, powders or deodorants to the vulval vaginal area.

■ Regular cleansing of the perineum is important, preferably by immersion in water or by spraying with warm water and washing with a bland soap. Perfumed soaps, oils, bubble baths or talcum powder may cause irritation and produce an allergic response.

■ After a bowel motion or micturition always wipe from the front of the perineum to the back to avoid invasion of harmful organisms.

■ During menstruation, change pads or tampons frequently and pay close attention to personal hygiene. Tampons with a build-up of menstrual products have been identified as the source of toxic shock syndrome, a serious form of septicaemia.

■ Seek medical advice when there is any type of discharge, malodour or dryness of the vagina, difficult or painful intercourse or bleeding other than regular periods.

■ Repeated infections may signal the need for oral medication together with counselling and treatment for the sexual partner in order to break the cycle of reinfection.

■ Recommend attendance at a genito-urinary clinic if necessary for confidential specialist advice.

■ Practise safer sex — use condoms.

■ Have a regular cervical smear test as recommended.

BACKGROUND INFORMATION

In women's reproductive years the vagina is slightly acidic, pH 3.5–4.5, which inhibits the growth of pathogenic organisms.

Following the menopause and loss of oestrogen, the vagina becomes more alkaline, the vaginal walls become thinner and secretions decrease, thus reducing natural protection. Vaginal dryness can make intercourse difficult and painful, but this is simply remedied by use of a water-based gel.

Alteration in the pH of the vagina upsets the natural balance and provides a more favourable environment for pathogenic organisms to flourish. Other causes of vulval irritation include glycosuria, skin infections such as psoriasis or scabies, infestation with pubic lice and allergy to toiletries.

Host defences are compromised by:
■ Diabetes or pregnancy   ■ Illness or malnutrition
■ Some oral contraceptives ■ Certain antibiotics
■ Steroid therapy   ■ Vaginal sprays or deodorants.

Pathogens can be introduced by:
■ Poor personal hygiene   ■ Sexual intercourse
■ Contamination from faeces ■ Douching
■ Vaginal intercourse following anal penetration
■ Unwashed vaginal inserts, sex toys
■ Neglected tampon or ring pessary
■ Mechanical contraceptive devices such as an IUD or cap.

The woman will complain of symptoms such as:
■ Vaginal discharge
■ Vulval irritation (pruritus)
■ Soreness, discomfort or burning
■ Reddening and swelling of vulval tissues
■ Sores or blisters on vulval area
■ Pain on intercourse (dyspareunia)
■ Urinary frequency, painful or burning micturition.

Common vaginal infections include:
■ Candidiasis (thrush)   ■ Trichomoniasis
■ Gonorrhoea   ■ Chlamydia
■ Herpes   ■ Human papilloma virus
■ Bacterial vaginitis.

Chronic cervicitis and post-menopausal vaginitis may also cause problems.

It is essential that the causative organism is identified, so a high vaginal swab may be necessary. The correct treatment is vital to prevent complications which may lead to infertility. If the GP is not knowledgeable about sexually transmitted diseases the client should be advised to go to a genito-urinary clinic. If a sexual partner appears to be infected or is acting as a reservoir for reinfection, he will also require treatment. If intercourse takes place, condom use should be advised, although medications may damage condoms or diaphragms.

NOW YOU SHOULD FEEL COMPETENT TO:

■ Advise clients and carers on the administration of vaginal medications

■ Administer vaginal medications

■ Offer advice on maintaining vaginal health.

EXTERNAL

WHO MAY PRESENT?

Clients after discharge by the orthopaedic team to continue management at home using external fixator systems for:
- Immobilisation of bones (without plaster) to allow fractures to unite
- Treatment to gain length in the long bones:
— Where there is inequality of leg length in children
— To gain height in cases of restricted growth (achondroplasia)
— To regain bone lost by trauma or non-union of fractures.

PRINCIPLES OF EXTERNAL FIXATION

- It can be used for fractures associated with severe soft-tissue injuries so that the wound can be accessed.
- The fracture is held by transfixing screws which pass through the bone above and below the fracture. These screws are attached to an external frame.
- This method is most commonly used for fractures of the tibia and the pelvis but may also be used for fractures of the femur, humerus and also for bones of the hand.
- Metal pins are fixed transversely into bone segments, then linked mechanically to external vertical struts or rods, providing a cantilever system.
- Alternatively, wires transfixed across bone are attached to an external ring resembling a wheel with spoke and a hub, as in the Ilizarov circular fixator.
- There are varying designs and configurations to suit differing treatment needs and anatomical sites. The weight is taken through the metal system, while maintaining approximation of bone ends securely.

BENEFITS

- It is a minimally invasive procedure, often an alternative to extensive surgery and the accompanying anaesthesia.
- It permits early ambulation and early weight-bearing, so reducing the complications of immobility.
- There is an opportunity to exercise adjacent joints and other muscles.
- It encourages blood flow to the healing area.
- Micromovement at the fracture site stimulates bone growth and healing of fractures.
- Early discharge home is possible to resume school or work.
- Clients have control and involvement in their care management.

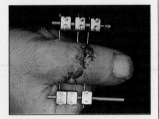

Fracture with external fixator on thumb

PIN SITE CARE

- There is no universally agreed method of managing pin site care and the nurse must follow the protocol determined by the orthopaedic team. If clients are to be self-caring, they should receive instruction and written information before discharge.
- If discharged into the care of the district nurse, ward staff must send detailed instructions on the pin site regime.
- Daily cleansing following scrupulous hand-washing is carried out by client or by a nurse wearing gloves.
- Instructions may include gently moving the skin to prevent it adhering to the metal pin. This permits tissue exudate to escape rather than getting trapped and setting up a moist site for infection.
- Using a sterile cotton bud, swab gently using the solution recommended in the protocol: either sterile water, cooled boiled water or a sachet of normal saline. Use one bud for each pin site and dry with another cotton bud.
- Additionally, the protocol may include cleaning around the metal pins using alcohol-impregnated wipes from a canister holder. A fresh wipe should be used for each pin.
- Dressings are not generally recommended around the pin site, as a clean site should be left dry and open to the air.
- It is not uncommon for crusts to develop around the pin site, and the nurse should refer back to the orthopaedic team, as there is controversy over whether to remove these or leave them in place.
- If there is oozing, cleanse twice daily using an aseptic technique with recommended solution and apply a non-adherent dressing.
- It is essential to watch for any sign of infection at the pin entry sites, as this could lead to osteomyelitis, that is, infection within the bone.
- Daily inspection of the pin sites should be carried out checking for redness, swelling, discharge (clear or purulent), offensive odour, pain, skin migrating up the pin like a 'tent', loosening of pins, sensation and movement of distal part of limb to confirm neurovascular status.
- If there are signs of infection a swab must be sent for culture and sensitivity. The client may require antibiotic treatment or, in more serious cases, removal or resiting of the pins may be necessary.

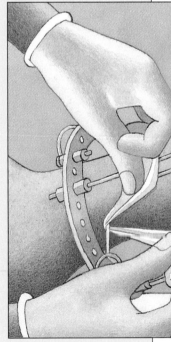

FIXATORS

CLIENT CARE

- While clients are generally happy to be able to continue treatment at home, they may need reassurance that they are making progress and managing their fixator satisfactorily.
- The client and carer may have difficulty adjusting to the altered body image and feel extremely conspicuous when out of doors. They should be encouraged to get involved in activities to offset social isolation.
- Clients need to adjust to a change in balance owing to the weight of the fixator. They must also avoid hitting their other leg or furniture, for fear of damaging these as well as disturbing the fixator system.
- Suitable clothing could include wide-legged tracksuit bottoms with an elasticated waist. These are easy to put on, large enough to conceal the fixator, warm and comfortable. It may be necessary to split the trousers and sew on tie-up strings. Shorts could be worn instead.
- When seated it is important to elevate and support the limb to avoid oedema.
- A bed cradle will protect the bedclothes and enable easier movement. A pillow between the legs can prevent damage to the other leg.
- The mobilisation regime must be adhered to, which may vary from wheelchair, ambulation on crutches — either non-weight-bearing or partial weight-bearing — to full ambulation without aids. Clients must be encouraged to exercise the adjacent joints and unaffected limbs.
- It is usually possible for clients to shower, perhaps with

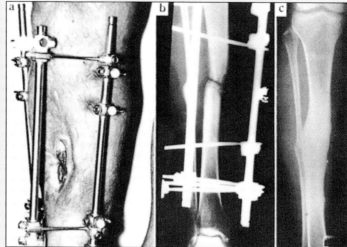

This patient had an open fracture with loss of skin (a,b). After debridement the fracture was held by external fixation. It went on to solid union (c). Reproduced with kind permission from Apley and Solomon's *Concise System of Orthopaedics and Fractures*

assistance, but it should be ensured that the pin sites are well dried afterwards.
- Clients on a leg-lengthening programme are given the responsibility of distracting the long bone four times a day. By moving a device the bone ends will be pulled apart gradually within telescopic rods paced so the leg is lengthened by 0.25mm at each turn. This regime must be rigidly adhered to in order to ensure the procedure's success. The majority of these clients are children or adolescents and, even though they will be under the supervision of the orthopaedic nurse specialist, all members of the family may need additional psychological and practical support and reassurance from the primary care team.

NOW YOU SHOULD BE AWARE OF:

- The needs of a client who is managing an external fixator at home
- The importance of identifying a link person in the orthopaedic team who can give specialist advice.

FURTHER READING
Apley, A.G., Solomon, L. *Concise System of Orthopaedics and Fractures* (2nd edn). Oxford: Butterworth-Heinemann, 1994.
Maher, A., Salmond, S., Pellino, T. *Orthopaedic Nursing*. Philadelphia: W.B. Saunders, 1994.
Wallis, S. Nursing care of skeletal pin sites. *Professional Nurse* 1991; **6:** 12, 715–720.

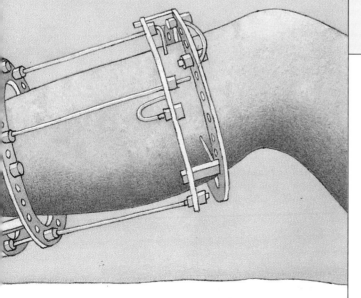

Cleaning the pin of an Ilizarov circular fixator

MOUTH CARE

WHO MAY PRESENT?

- Clients with mouth infection, ulceration or bleeding, associated with dehydration, debilitating disease or radiotherapy to the head and neck area and clients who are mouth breathing or on oxygen therapy
- Clients affected by any illness, drug regime or surgery inducing nausea, vomiting or anorexia. This can reduce the desire to eat or drink and will affect oral hygiene and the condition of the mouth
- Clients receiving cytotoxic chemotherapy. They can be subject to severe ulceration, for example, doxorubicin and drugs that are folic acid antagonists, such as methotrexate. Part of the rescue regime is to restore the depletion by giving folinic acid, but the client should be forewarned to be alert to the possibility of ulcer formation and stomatitis
- Clients who are immunocompromised or immunosuppressed, owing to drug treatment or HIV/AIDS. They are prone to mouth ulcers, gum bleeding and *Herpes simplex* infection
- Clients on drugs such as antidepressants and antihistamines which cause dryness of the mouth, phenytoin which causes gum hypertrophy and antibiotics which permit the proliferation of *Candida albicans* leading to candidiasis (thrush infection)
- Any client finding it difficult to maintain mouth hygiene.

ASSESSMENT

- The mouth is a useful indicator of both well-being and ill health or debility. Thorough examination of the mouth may reveal abnormalities, infection or malignancy that may be resolved by early detection and treatment.
- A healthy mouth should be moist, pink, clean and free from odour and pain or discomfort.
- Discuss the client's general condition, diet and fluid intake, normal oral hygiene regime and periodic dental checks.
- Assess the client's ability to achieve adequate mouth care and offer appropriate help and advice to the client and/or the carer to maximise his or her independence.
- Examine the mouth with gloved hands, using a pen torch, observing for problem areas such as:
  — Dry, cracked lips especially in the corners of the mouth
  — *Herpes simplex* viral infection (cold sores) on the lips or inside the mouth. This is amenable to treatment with anti-viral preparations such as acyclovir cream. The client should be advised to take care not to spread infection further on the lips, mouth, up to the eyes or to other people
  — A dry mouth and coated tongue, which is a sign of general dehydration and/or lack of oral fluids and/or lack of oral hygiene
  — Areas of soreness or irritation, swelling, encrustation or ulceration
  — Bleeding gums after brushing, which may indicate gum disease or a low platelet count
  — Patches of white indicating candida. This is amenable to treatment with anti-fungal preparations such as nystatin
  — Obvious dental caries or poorly fitting dentures, which can cause soreness and are open sites for infection
  — Glossitis, a shiny, smooth, red tongue which may indicate pernicious anaemia and vitamin B_{12} deficiency
  — Halitosis or odorous breath
  — Brittle, dry, dark, jagged and uneven teeth in elderly people. Gums lose vascularity and tissue elasticity then retract, exposing the part of the tooth not protected by enamel. This is an obvious site for infection and sensitivity. Dentures may also need adjustment

FLOSSING

- Interdental care is important to ensure cleansing between the teeth and removal of food debris. Daily flossing will minimise the build-up of plaque and tartar, especially where teeth and gums meet.
- Where appropriate, gloves should be worn. A flossing strip is wound round the two middle fingers and pulled tense between the thumb and index fingers.
- The floss is passed into the gaps between the teeth up to the gum margin, moved gently up and down, in and out in a seesaw action. A clean section is wound on each time as the client or carer proceeds around the mouth.
- Flossing may be problematic for people with difficulty with fine hand movements or vision. Flossing swords provide a floss under tension and may be easier to use.

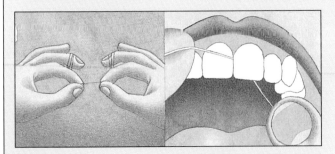
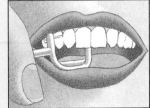

BRUSHING

- The mouth should be cleaned after taking food. Three times a day and before retiring to bed is advisable.
- If the client is debilitated recommend that he or she takes plenty of oral fluids to counteract dehydration and keep the mouth moist and fresh. Alternatively, suggest the client sucks ice chips, either plain or flavoured; this will stimulate saliva flow. An atomised water spray is useful for clients who are disinclined to drink.
- If clients are prone to ulceration or gingivitis it is important to use a small-headed, soft-bristled toothbrush that will not be abrasive to gums and soft tissues. Often a baby's brush is most suitable.
- If a client lacks manipulative skills, a large-handled toothbrush may be useful or one with an angled head; also a battery-operated toothbrush and mechanical toothpaste squeezer. A triple-headed toothbrush is effective in reaching all three surfaces of the teeth simultaneously.
- The nurse should put on gloves and protect the client with a towel, then load the brush with toothpaste and help the client do as much as he or she can. She should hold the brush at an angle of 45 degrees with the bristles towards the edge of the gums and make short, gentle, horizontal strokes, moving in zig-zag fashion from gum to crown on the outer surfaces of the teeth.

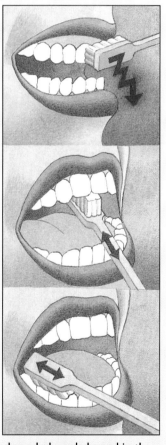

- To clean inner surfaces, tilt the brush to get behind the teeth and use short back and forth strokes. Clean the biting surfaces of both upper and lower teeth by brushing back and forth.
- The complete brushing cycle should continue for a minimum of two minutes. One thorough brushing is more beneficial than frequent but cursory brushing.
- Dentures must be removed regularly and cleaned in the same way with a toothbrush and denture cream. Abrasive soaking agents are not recommended. The gums and mouth of the edentulous client should be cleaned using brush and paste, followed by a rinsing agent.
- If a client cannot tolerate toothbrush cleaning or cannot hold his or her mouth open, the nurse or carer should use a gloved finger wrapped with cotton wool or a soft piece of sponge dipped in mouthwash to clean the surfaces of the teeth and around the mouth.

WASHING OUT THE MOUTH

- Clients should be offered clean water to provide several rinses to swish around the whole of the mouth, with a bowl provided to spit out the fluid.
- Some clients, particularly those who are very sick, frail or those who have to remain lying down, may find it easier to suck the rinsing water through a straw, a feeder cup or beaker and spit it out by the same route.
- If a client cannot sip but is able to spit fluid out, the nurse could insert oral fluids into the cheek pouch via a syringe. She should wear gloves to do this.
- For clients prone to mouth ulceration, especially those on cytotoxic chemotherapy, a mouthwash is recommended, such as Oraldene, Difflam or Corsodyl. All these are available on prescription or as over-the-counter preparations. Alternatively a thymol solution may be used.
- A mouthwash of chlorhexidine gluconate 1% is effective in reducing plaque build-up and has a significant anti-microbial action if used after teeth cleaning and rinsed around the mouth for a full minute.

COMPLETION

- Wearing gloves, inspect the mouth for sores, ulceration or bleeding.
- Apply any prescribed creams, suspensions or lotions.
- Replace dentures and wipe around the client's mouth if he or she cannot do this alone.
- Moisten the lips with a fine film of soft paraffin, vaseline or a proprietary lip salve with a flavour agreeable to the client.
- Remove the towel and clear away equipment, rinsing the toothbrush well. Remove gloves and wash your hands.
- Leave the client sitting or lying in a comfortable position, with instructions on fluid intake. If appropriate, fluids should be left within reach of the client.
- Document the procedure. If necessary refer the client to GP or dentist. Note that a dental domiciliary service is available for housebound people.

NOW YOU SHOULD FEEL COMPETENT TO:

- Advise clients and carers on an effective daily oral hygiene regime
- Advise and help clients who need assistance with mouth care.

FURTHER READING
Crosby, C. Method in mouth care. *Nursing Times* 1989; 85: 35, 38–41.
Heals, D. A key to well-being: oral hygiene in patients with advanced cancer. *Professional Nurse* 1993; **8**: 6, 391–398.

BANDAGING

WHO MAY PRESENT?

Clients needing a bandage:
- To hold a dressing securely in place, especially in the case of those people who cannot tolerate adhesive tapes on their skin
- To protect a wound site
- As protection for clothing, bedding or furnishings if there is discharge from wounds, or after application of ointments or lotions
- To give light support to a joint and limit swelling
  - After a soft tissue injury, for example, a ligamentous sprain of the ankle
  - Following the removal of a plaster of Paris cast, for example, a Colles' wrist fracture
  - Following the removal of sutures after surgery, for example, carpal tunnel compression.

CHOICE OF BANDAGE

It should be:
- Appropriate for the intended purpose
- Comfortable and acceptable to the client
- Easy to apply, fit securely and not be too bulky
- Cost-effective and available
- The correct size: roller bandages should be 2.5cm for fingers; 5–7.5cm for hands, arms and feet; 7.5–10cm for legs.

CLIENT CHECKLIST

- Ensure that the client understands the purpose of the bandage, how long it is to remain in place, when it will be removed and by whom. May he or she remove it and can the client or carer reapply it? What should be done if it becomes loose or uncomfortable or exerts pressure? Discuss what can be done by the client or carer if it gets grubby — for instance, can it be washed?
- The distal part of limb or digit should be checked regularly to ensure that the circulation and nerve supply are not impeded; this involves checking for good colour, warmth, sensation and movement.
- Any itching, irritation or burning may signal skin damage and a developing pressure sore. This is especially a hazard in the presence of swelling or oedema, poor-quality skin and bony prominences such as malleoli and the tibial crest. The bandage should be taken off, the skin should be examined, details documented in the patient's notes and the bandage reapplied.
- Confirm any additional instructions to the client, such as keeping the limb elevated when not in use or wearing a sling.
- The client should be advised on suitable clothing. Tights and socks will give further protection to lower limb wounds and keep the bandage clean. When feet and legs are bandaged, supportive wide, flat footwear is recommended. The client should ensure that the bandage does not get wet.

TYPES OF BANDAGES

BANDAGES FOR THE RETENTION OF DRESSINGS
- **Open-weave cotton**
  These hold reasonably well but have no conforming properties, so they may prove unsuitable for more active clients.
- **Conformable types**
  Cotton, viscose or rayon are lightweight. They provide good hold and allow for some movement of a joint because the two-way stretch permits conformity to bodily contours. They do not provide significant pressure and should not be applied when support is required. The newer cohesive bandages have auto-adhesive properties so that they adhere to themselves but not to skin or clothing. This helps with closure after bandaging and also limits slipping during wearing.
- **Tubular stockinette**
  This is quick and easy to apply as long as the nurse has access to the range of applicators and bandages.
- **Tubular elastic net**
  This is ideal for dressings covering large areas. It is cool,

does not fray, allows visibility and ease of access. It is easy to apply, good for limbs but especially useful for head, thorax and trunk. Ready-to-wear garments are also available, as vest or pants.

BANDAGES TO PROVIDE LIGHT SUPPORT
- **Elastic crêpe**
  These provide retention and control of tissue without the application of compression and should be stretched to one-third of their length to give adequate support. They can be washed and will regain a degree of elasticity for reapplication a few times. (Unless there is a lot of wound exudate, a crêpe should not be used for dressing retention, as it is over 10 times the cost of the cheapest retention product.) Crêpe bandage is *not* suitable for applying compression in the treatment of venous leg ulcers.
- **Elasticated tubular support**
  This ensures even support and pressure over the affected area. Apply with or without an applicator.

ROLLER BANDAGE TECHNIQUE

- The nurse and client should be seated facing one another to limit static back strain. The limb should be supported and, if swelling is present or there is the possibility it will develop, elevate the limb before bandaging is begun.
- Always work from the distal end of the limb to the proximal (ascending towards the body). This promotes venous return, which minimises oedema and circulatory impairment. Work from the medial to lateral side of the limb (inwards to outwards) towards an unencumbered area.
- Hold the bandage with the roll (or head) uppermost and feed from the loose end (or tail) with the other hand. It is ideal to work with the roll in your dominant hand; however, for a left limb, hold the roll in the right hand; for the right limb, hold it in the left hand.
- Do not begin or end a bandage over a wound site. Start with one firm turn to anchor the bandage. Then continue working up the limb in spiral fashion, moulding to contours. Successive turns should overlap two-thirds of the preceding turn. Ensure that tension is applied firmly and evenly to maintain a regular pressure, especially with a support bandage. If the bandage is too loose, it will be ineffective and fall down. If it is too tight, it could impair circulation and nerve conduction and may cause skin necrosis, leading to a pressure sore.
- If a joint is to be enclosed, the technique is a figure of eight, radiating from the central point, winding above and below sequentially. This permits some movement at the joint.
- Complete the bandage with a circumferential turn ending on the lateral side of the limb. Affix it securely either with adhesive tape, bandage clip or auto-adhesion. Clients may wish to use a safety pin, but this is to be discouraged as it may damage the skin and tear clothes.

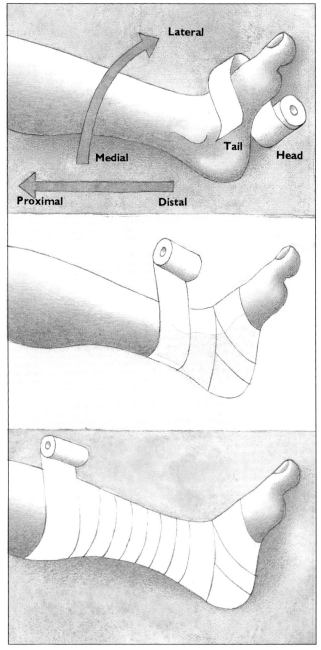

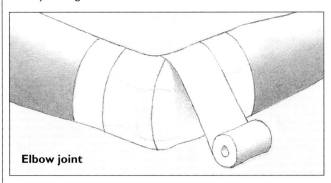

Elbow joint

NOW YOU SHOULD FEEL COMPETENT TO:

- Apply roller bandages for retention of dressings or light support
- Understand what complications to observe for and to advise clients who need to wear a bandage.

Note
This article does not address the application of elastic adhesive strapping for strong support or compression bandaging for venous leg ulcers; nor does it explain tubular bandage technique.

FURTHER READING
Thomas, S. Bandages and bandaging: the science behind the art. *Care Science and Practice* 1990; **8**: 2, 55–60.
Walsh, M., Orford, J., Love, C., Jamieson, E.L. Back to the art of bandaging. *Nursing Times* 1989; **85**: 27, Suppl. 1–15.

GASTROSTOMY

WHO MAY PRESENT?

- Clients requiring supplementary nutrition or regular small-dose feeding by infusion, as in malabsorption syndromes (although there must be adequate, intestinal absorptive capacity), debilitation or malnutrition, short bowel, inflammatory bowel or Crohn's disease
- Clients requiring complete dietary replacement when the oral route is inaccessible, such as obstruction owing to burns, injury or carcinoma or when they are unable to swallow as in stroke, motor neurone disease, muscular dystrophy or multiple sclerosis
- Carers/parents and clients who can manage their gastrostomy at home and who need support, advice or assistance.

BACKGROUND INFORMATION

- Gastrostomy is a direct method of providing nutrition that has advantages for long-term feeding in preference to a nasogastric tube or parenteral infusion. It is unobtrusive, more socially acceptable and does not cause pharyngeal erosion or discomfort or damage veins. Feeds can be administered slowly overnight or in bolus form, leaving long periods in the day free of feeding. An ambulatory backpack and pump system gives discreet feeding which allows the client to pursue uninterrupted activities at work or school.
- Many clients are able to manage their own gastrostomy feeding regime or carers can be supported in doing so. The nurse must be aware of local arrangements for services with regard to provision and funding of feeding bags/infusion sets, pumps and feeds, maintainance, instruction and training for staff and carers.
- The most common method is using a percutaneous endoscopic gastrostomy (PEG) tube which is drawn out through the stomach wall and abdominal wall, positioned using a gastroscope with the client under general anaesthetic or sedation. This tube may remain in place between one and three years. Within the stomach the tube is held in place by devices such as a retainer disc or a retention balloon. On the outside, close to the abdominal wall, is a guard or fixation device which will prevent the tube being sucked inwards. It also enables the tube to turn through 90°, to lie flat to the skin, yet remain patent without kinking.
- A replacement gastrostomy tube with an internal balloon may be inserted into the stomach through an established stoma. Once in place the balloon is inflated with sterile water or saline. A replacement catheter will last between three and six months before it needs changing, and in some instances this may be undertaken by an experienced district nurse. Tubes with an internal shield need replacement by endoscopy.
- A button-style gastrostomy lies flush to the abdominal wall with a closure, giving a cosmetically neat appearance and without having a tube dangling between feeds.
- Systems will have a two-way connection with stopper closures that permits direct feeding and has a side port for syringe flushing with water or for liquid medication.

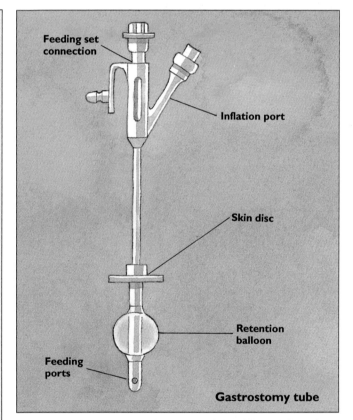

Feeding set connection

Inflation port

Skin disc

Retention balloon

Feeding ports

Gastrostomy tube

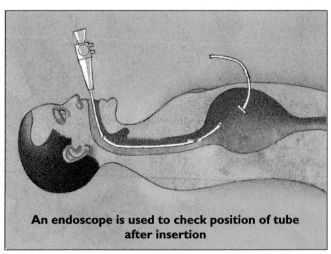

An endoscope is used to check position of tube after insertion

ADMINISTERING FEEDS

A gastrostomy feeding regime will be established by the nutrition team at the hospital and instruction given about the type of feed and the daily amount required. In consultation with the client, the method and timing of administration will be agreed, whether bolus, intermittent feeds, gravity drip or via pump, during the day or overnight. The container for overnight feeding should be large enough to avoid the need for changing or refilling during the night.

There are various proprietary feeds on the market that provide total replacement nutrition and these are available on prescription. Different types cater for special needs, such as high-fibre, gluten-free, high-calorie, high-protein. There may also be a selection of flavours.

The prescribed type and amount of feed is prepared at body temperature. The procedure is as follows:

- Explain to the client that a feed is to be given and, if possible, place him or her in a position to elevate the head and chest to avoid gastro-oesophageal reflux.
- Take the giving set and feed bag, ensuring that the regulator switch is closed off.
- Pour the feed through the porthole on the side of the bag, then press the porthole cap securely to close, or attach prepared bag or bottle-feed. Hang the bag on the drip stand and squeeze the drip chamber to fill it half full.
- Flush about 50ml of water in through the side of a Y-connection attached to the gastrostomy tube.
- Remove the Luer cap of the giving set and allow feed to fill the tube, thus ensuring that the client is not given air which might cause discomfort. Connect the giving set to the main route of the gastrostomy tube.
- If the client requires a regular metered dose of feed with a controlled administration, the infusion tube should be passed through a pump.
- When the feed is completed, once again flush the gastrostomy tube syringing with about 50ml of water.
- Liquid medication can be added to the feed if it is stable or it can be administered via a side Y-connection.
- If the gastrostomy tube gets blocked it can be cleared by flushing with effervescent soda water.
- The bag and infusion set should be changed every 24 hours, as there may be a build-up of harmful pathogens within the system.

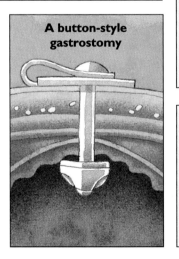

Tube lying flush against abdominal wall

A button-style gastrostomy

CARE OF THE STOMA

- Initially, when the fixation device is in place, the gastrostomy site is treated as a surgical wound with the appropriate dressing if necessary.
- Once the stoma is established and the tissues have healed, no dressing should be applied to the site, as the build-up of mucus will create a soggy environment, predisposing to infection, excoriation and overgranulation.
- A small amount of mucous secretion can be expected from the tract, but the gastric contents should not leak.
- Dismantle the fixation device/guard and slide it up around the tube.
- Observe the stoma for redness, irritation, excoriation, gastric leakage or infection.
- If necessary, the stoma site should be washed with warm soapy water, rinsed and dried thoroughly. A light dusting of non-perfumed talc may then be applied.
- Rotate the tube a full circle on its axis within the stoma, to dislodge any exudate and prevent pressure necrosis from the internal retainer.
- Reassemble the fixation device.
- Daily wiping of the stoma site and guard with water and a swab should be sufficient.

CLIENT CARE

- Clients must be supported in this unnatural way of feeding. Because they may not wish to join the family at mealtimes, other opportunities for regular family socialisation should be created.
- If the client is able to drink, fluids should be encouraged to keep the mouth fresh and to stimulate saliva production.
- Regular teeth cleaning and rinsing is important; mouth care must be given for the dependent client.
- If conscious but unable to swallow, the client may be able to rinse the mouth with tasty fluids or to chew foods, then eject them from the mouth.
- Clients or carers should report any diarrhoea, constipation, abdominal distension, cramps, nausea or dehydration; and patients should be weighed regularly. These factors may indicate a need to alter the feeding regime or diet.
- Clients can take a bath or shower as normal providing the gastrostomy connections are closed and the stoma site is dried well.
- Clients should have a contact person in the nutrition team who can advise over any difficulties with the diet.

NOW YOU SHOULD BE AWARE OF:

- The needs and care of a client with a gastrostomy.

Magic Time

Activity Book 1

Robin Davis • Günter Gerngross • Christian Holzmann • Herbert Puchta

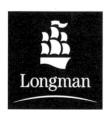

Longman

Pearson Education Limited
Edinburgh Gate, Harlow,
Essex. CM20 2JE England
and Associated Companies throughout the world

www.longman.com

First published by Langenscheidt - Verlag Ges. m.b.H., Vienna 1993
The edition published by Longman Group Ltd. 1995
Eighteenth impression 2010
ISBN 978-0-582-24744-4

Printed in Malaysia, PPSB
Set in 9/11pt Helvetica

The Publishers' policy is to use paper manufactured from sustainable forests.

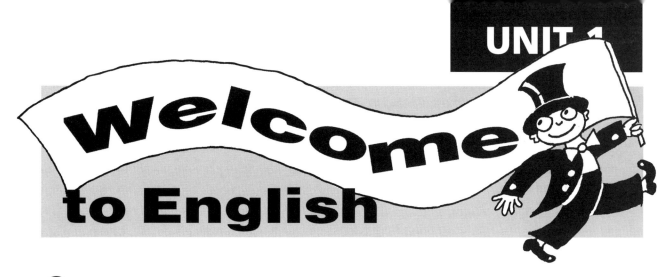

Welcome to English

1 *Write the words in the boxes.*

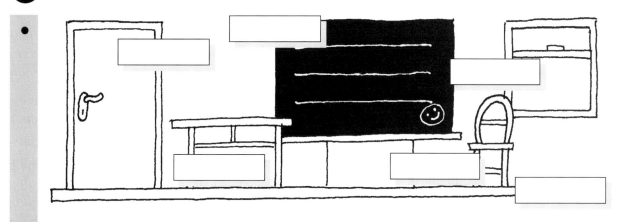

2 *Write the numbers.*

★ xsi __six__   nien _____   evnse _____

hitge _____   otw _____   eno _____

tehre _____   rofu _____   vife _____

3 *What is the next number? Write it out.*

■ 2   4   6 __eight__   1 3 2 4 3 _____

7   6   5 _____   12 1 11 2 10 _____

2   5   8 _____   1 6 2 7 3 _____

4 *Fill in the missing words.*

• one __mountain bike__   six _____

two _____   seven _____

three _____   eight _____

four _____   nine _____

five _____   ten _____

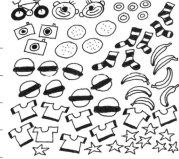

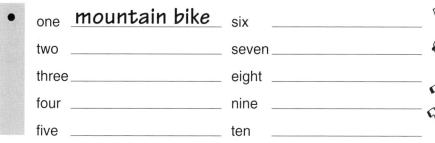

5 *Use your colour pens to draw the goblin's dream.*

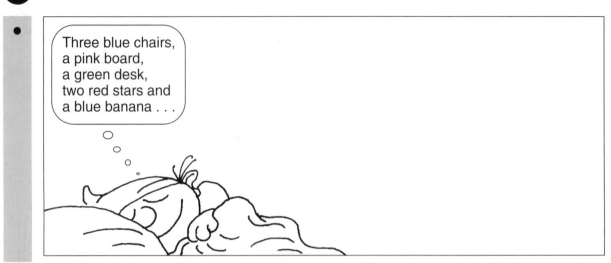

Three blue chairs,
a pink board,
a green desk,
two red stars and
a blue banana . . .

6 *Fill in the right numbers. Write the sentences under the pictures.*

3	Touch the floor.
	Sit down.
	Point at the window.
	Stand up.
	Turn around.
	Point at the board.
	Touch your desk.
	Walk round your chair.
	Point at the door.
	Jump.

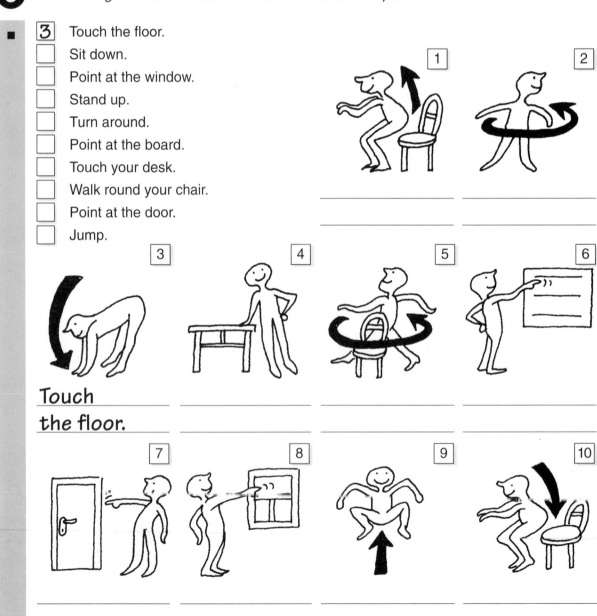

Touch
the floor.

4

Wordfields

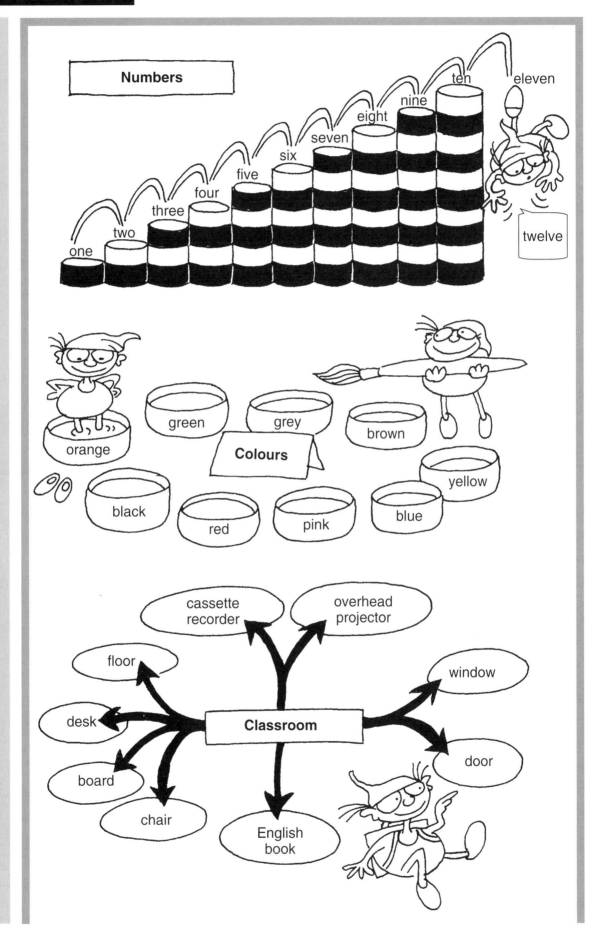

Numbers

one, two, three, four, five, six, seven, eight, nine, ten, eleven, twelve

Colours

orange, green, grey, brown, yellow, black, red, pink, blue

Classroom

cassette recorder, overhead projector, floor, window, desk, door, board, chair, English book

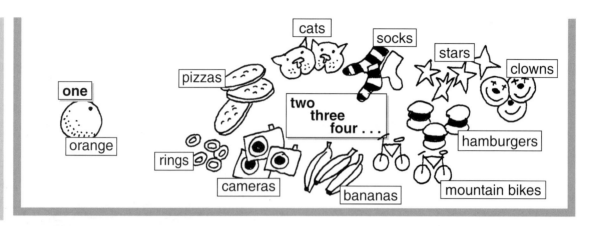

one
orange
pizzas
cats
socks
stars
clowns
two
three
four . . .
hamburgers
rings
cameras
bananas
mountain bikes

Words in context

Write the words in your language here:

6 telephone number   What's your telephone number?
Thank you.

8 ready   Are you ready?
stand up
turn around
touch   Touch the floor.
walk round   Walk round your chair.
point at   Point at the board.
jump
sit down

10 tell   Tell me.
back   I'll write it on your back.
that   That's it.

11 colour   Colour the stars yellow.

12 colour   What colour is your mountain bike?
it's (= it is)   It's blue.

13 goblin
midnight
give   Give me the blue paint.
now
Let's (= let us) go.

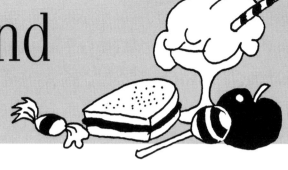

UNIT 2

Sweets and snacks

Revision

1 **Grammar**

Fill in the missing words.

one _____

three _____

two _____

five _____

one _____

four _____

2 *Sort out the words.*

green ICE CREAM Chewing gum board window

yellow chair pink GREY BLACK

desk SWEET toffee

white lolly floor fruit gum

cassette recorder red CHOCOLATE door

colours

classroom

sweets

7

3 *Fill in:* **a – an**

an apple _____ orange T-shirt _____ banana _____ chair _____ white desk

_____ toffee _____ yellow floor _____ orange _____ camera _____ sandwich

_____ lolly _____ ice cream _____ fruit gum _____ pink lolly _____ red apple

4 *Number the sentences in the right order to make two dialogues.*

☐ What flavour?
☐ Yes, please.
1 Ice cream?
☐ Strawberry.

☐ Yes?
☐ 5-7-3-2-1-1-4.
1 Kate?
☐ What's your telephone number?

5 *Complete.*

c**hewing** g**um** _____, Mark?

Yes, p_____.

H_____ you are.

T_____ y_____.

Do you w_____ o_____, Sylvia?

W_____ f_____ is it?

S_____.

No, t_____ y_____.
I h_____ s_____.

6 *Write the correct numbers in the boxes. Write the sentences under the pictures.*

| 1 | 2 | ☐ Pay for it. |

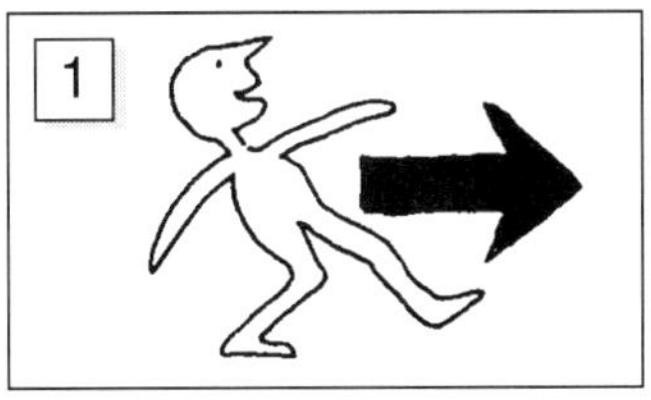

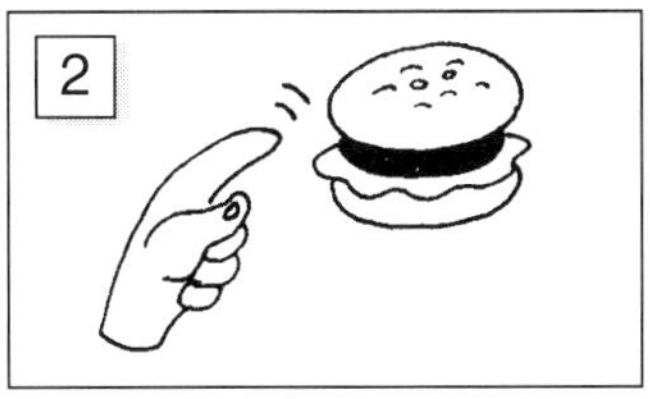

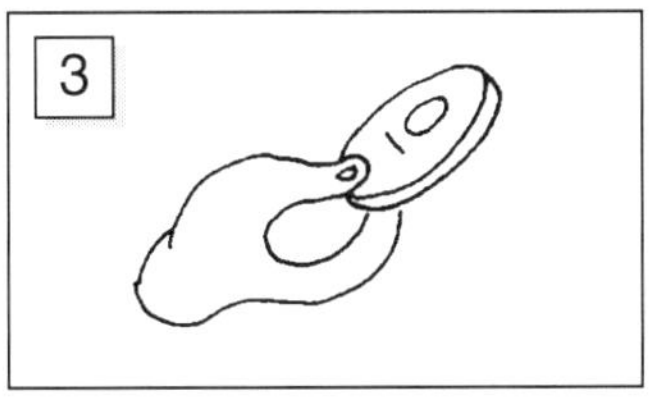

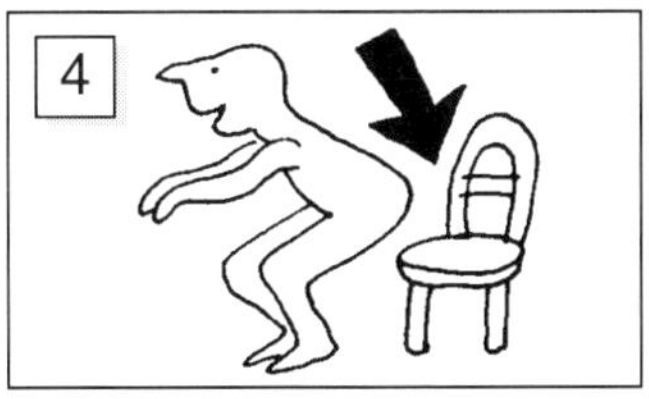

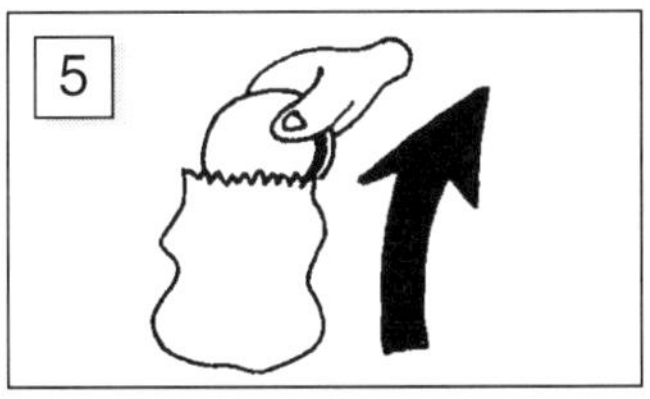

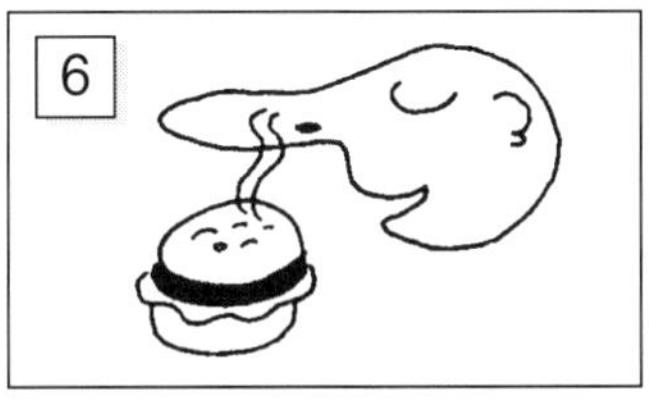

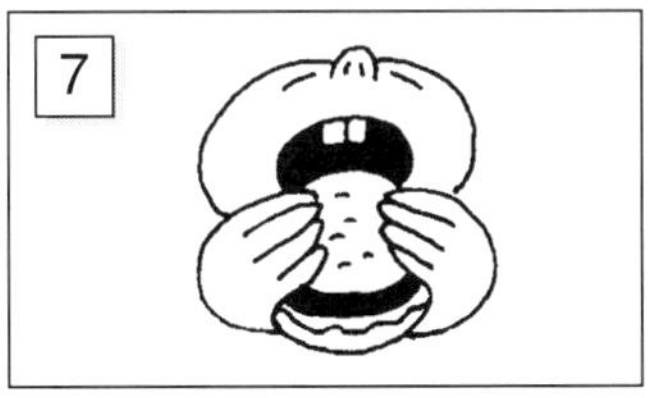

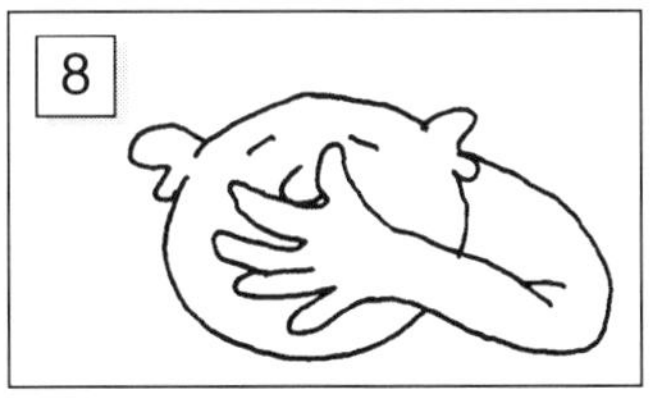

☐ Go to a snack bar.

☐ Sit down.

| 3 | 4 | ☐ Order a hamburger. |

☐ Smell it.

| 5 | 6 | ☐ Wipe the ketchup off your face. |

☐ Take a bite of the hamburger.

☐ Take out the hamburger.

| 7 | 8 |

7 *Write the questions and answers.*

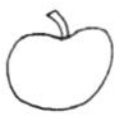

Do you want an apple? ☺ Yes, please.

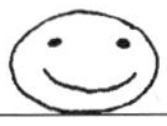

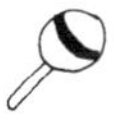

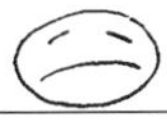

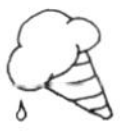

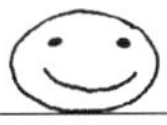

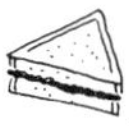

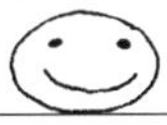

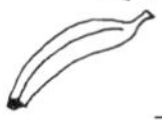

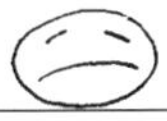

☹

☺

☺

☹

8 *Write the dialogues.*

Do you like _____ | _____ | _____

_____ | _____ | _____

_____ | _____ | _____

_____

Wordfields

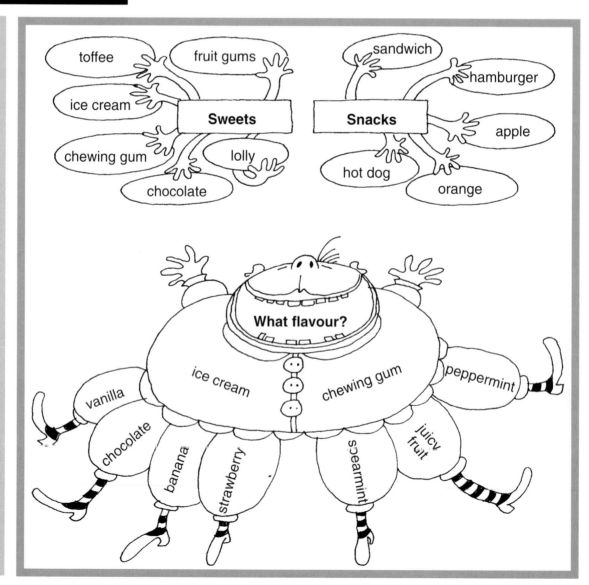

toffee   fruit gums   sandwich   hamburger

ice cream   **Sweets**   **Snacks**   apple

chewing gum   lolly   hot dog   orange

chocolate

What flavour?

ice cream   chewing gum   peppermint

vanilla

chocolate   banana   strawberry   spearmint   juicy fruit

10

Words in context

*Write the words in
your language here:*

3   Yummy.

Ouch! [aʊtʃ]

what   What do you want?

4   flavour   What flavour?

5   want   Do you want a lolly?

Yes, please.

No, thank you.

6   Here you are.

hate   I hate peppermint.

7   hungry   Are you hungry?

snack bar   Go to the snack bar.

order   Order a hamburger.

pay   Pay for it.

take out   Take out the hamburger.

smell   Smell the hamburger.

a bite   Take a bite of the hamburger.

face

wipe off   Wipe the ketchup off your face.

9   like   I like muesli.

coffee

milk

yoghurt

10   Do you like . . .?

Yes, I do.

No, I don't (= do not).

11

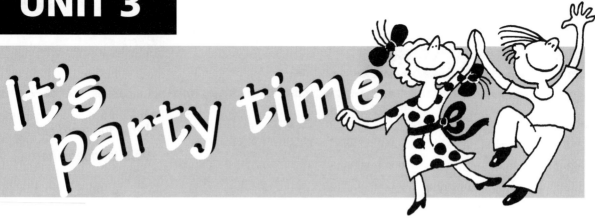

UNIT 3

It's party time

Revision

1 **Grammar**

Fill in: **a – an**

_____ cake _____ exercise book _____ nice party _____ pencil case

_____ idea _____ good idea _____ English book _____ very good pizza

2 **Grammar**

Fill in the questiions and/or the answers.

Do you like bananas? ☺ <u>**Yes, I do.**</u>

_____ ? ☹ No, I don't.

_____ ? ☹ _____

_____ ? ☺ _____

3 **Grammar**

Add an **s** *where it is needed.*

five schoolbag **s** a cold orange juice____ two exercise book____ five apple____

a good film____ a telephone number____ ten fruit gum____ two goblin____

4 *Fill in the words from the box.*

On her way home from _____ Sandra meets her _____ Mary.

"Let's have a _____ ," Mary says. "A _____ ?" Sandra asks.

"Yes, let's have a party. A party is great _____ ."

Sandra and Mary meet Tom, Frank, Susan and Bob.

And they all _____ to the party. The party _____ at six o'clock

in Mary's _____ . They _____ all very happy.

"Thank _____ , Mary. The party is great," they say.

| school |
| is |
| come |
| are |
| party |
| garden |
| you |
| friend |
| fun |
| party |

5 *Number the sentences in the right order to make two dialogues.*

☐ Yes, it's the beginning of the school year.
1 Hallo, Sarah.
☐ A party?
☐ Good idea.
☐ Let's have a party.
☐ Hallo, Tom.

☐ How are you, Pam?
☐ Oh, good.
☐ Hallo, Mrs Clark
☐ I'm fine, thank you.
☐ The party is great fun.
1 Hallo, Pam.

6 *Fill in the words from the box.*

Sarah, Cathy, Rick and Tina _____ Pam.

They _____ Jim, they _____ Tony,

they _____ Monica, and they _____ Jenny.

And they all _____ to the _____ .

At five o'clock Sarah's _____ is full of her friends.

The party is _____ fun!

meet
great
party
meet
garden
meet
meet
meet
come

7 *Can you complete the words on the stickers?*
The missing letters are in the grey circle.

GOOD I _ _ A!

L _ _ ' S
H _ _ E A
P _ _ _ Y.

I ' _ F _ _ _ E.

I _ ' S
G _ _ _ _ T F _ N!

M U
D R
T E Ø I
V E N
A E
Ø T R T
E
A A

8 *Fill in: **am – is – are***

_____ you alright, Sandra? Yes, great.

The party _____ at five o'clock.

Sarah _____ on her way home from school.

The party _____ great fun. I _____ happy.

Monica, Jim, Tina, Tony, Rick, Pam and Cathy _____ in Sarah's garden.

Sarah and Frank, _____ you two okay?

13

9 *Join the questions to the correct answers.*

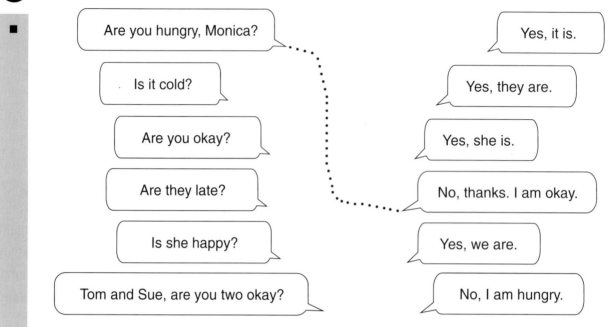

Are you hungry, Monica?

Is it cold?

Are you okay?

Are they late?

Is she happy?

Tom and Sue, are you two okay?

Yes, it is.

Yes, they are.

Yes, she is.

No, thanks. I am okay.

Yes, we are.

No, I am hungry.

10 *Write out who the things belong to.*

Example:

Rick's sharpeners are number one.

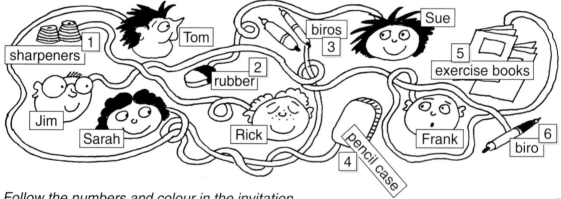

Tom
biros 3
Sue
sharpeners 1
5 exercise books
2 rubber
Jim
Sarah
Rick
pencil case 4
Frank
biro 6

11 *Follow the numbers and colour in the invitation.*

1 blue
2 red
3 green
4 brown
5 pink
6 yellow

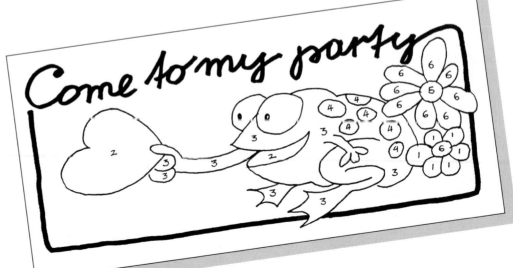

14

Wordfields

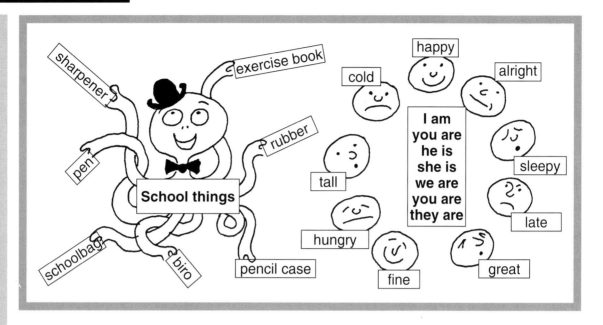

Words in context

Write the words in your language here:

3

on her way	Sarah is on her way home.
meets	Sarah meets Jenny.
friend	
her	Sarah and her friend
let's	
says	"Let's have a party", Sarah says.
asks	"A party?" Sarah asks.
the beginning of the school year	
idea	That's a good idea.
they all	They all come to the party.
at five o'clock	
full of	Sarah's garden is full of her friends.

7

I'm (= I am)	Hallo, I'm Mary.
song	Let's sing a song.
cake	Thank you for the cake.
lovely	It's lovely.
cut	Let's cut the cake.
what a	What a great party!

8 How are you?

9 very   It's a very good book.

15

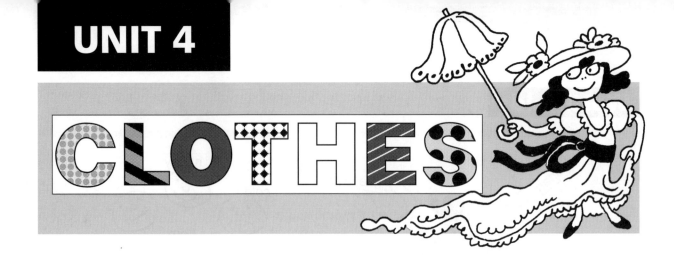

UNIT 4

CLOTHES

1 *Work with a partner.*

Partner A: Ask the prices.
Partner B: Look at the box below. Tell your partner the prices.

Textbook ▸ 7

Your partner says:

You say:

| How much | **is** the T-shirt | ? |

| **are** the jeans |

It's five pounds forty.

They're twenty-nine pounds ninety.

T-shirt	£ 5.40	sweater	£ 47.00
jeans	£ 29.90	socks	£ 2.70
trainers	£ 62.00	jacket	£ 39.90

2 *Work with a partner.*

Partner B: Ask for the prices. Fill them in.
Partner A: Look in your textbook.

Textbook ▸ 8

You say:

Your partner says:

| How much | **is** the ... | ? |

| **are** the ... |

It's...

They're...

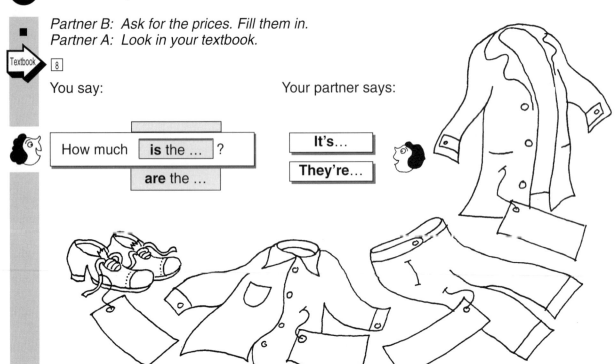

16

3 *Fill in the figures or the words.*

eleven (**11**)   seventeen (   )   _____ (24)

_____ (12)   eighteen (   )   twenty-five   (   )

thirteen (   )   nineteen (   )   _____ (26)

_____ (14)   twenty-one (   )   _____ (27)

_____ (15)   _____ (22)   twenty-eight (   )

sixteen (   )   _____ (23)   twenty-nine   (   )

4 *Do the sums and write the answers.*

You say: Eleven plus nineteen is thirty.
          Twenty-seven minus . . .

11 + 19 = **thirty** _____

27 – 16 = _____   16 + 37 = _____

86 – 46 = _____   38 + 62 = _____

41 + 28 = _____   96 – 73 = _____

5 *Write the questions and the answers.*

Example:

How much is the dress?   It's twenty-three pounds fifty.

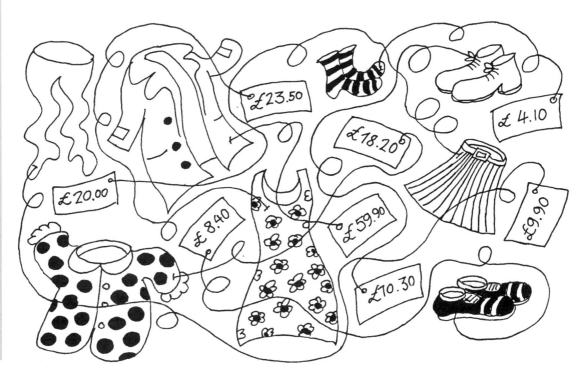

6 *Fill in the missing words.*

Do you _____ a toffee?   Yes, please.

_____ is your telephone number?   6-7-8-1-2-0.

What _____ is it?   Peppermint.

What _____ is her skirt?   White.

Let's _____ a party.   Good idea.

_____ are you, Monica?   Fine, thanks.

Can I _____ your pencil?   Yes, here you are.

What colour _____ her shoes?   Red.

Wordfields

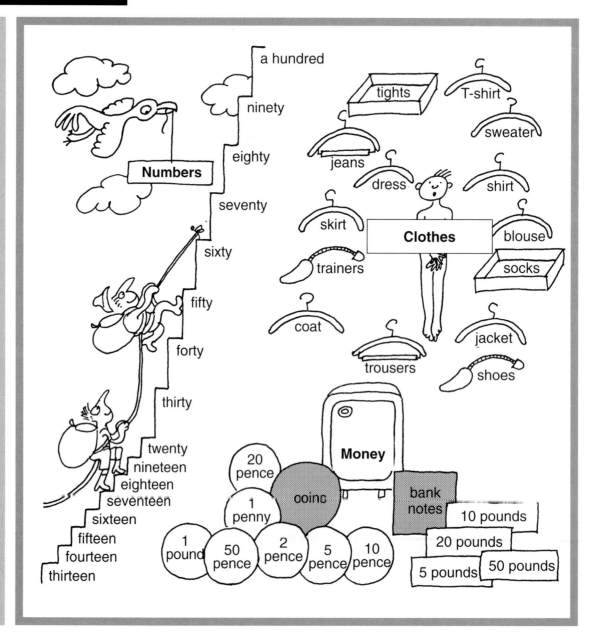

a hundred
ninety
eighty
seventy
sixty
fifty
forty
thirty
twenty
nineteen
eighteen
seventeen
sixteen
fifteen
fourteen
thirteen

Numbers

tights
T-shirt
jeans
sweater
dress
shirt
skirt
trainers
blouse
socks
coat
jacket
trousers
shoes

Clothes

Money

20 pence
1 penny
coins
bank notes
10 pounds
20 pounds
5 pounds
50 pounds
1 pound
50 pence
2 pence
5 pence
10 pence

Words in context

4	rainbow	How much is the T-shirt with the rainbow on it?	
	butterfly	How much is the T-shirt with the butterfly on it?	
	beautiful	Her dress is beautiful.	

6	price		
	excuse me		
	How much is the sweater?		
	It's five pounds twenty.		
	How much are the shoes?		
	They're twenty pounds.		
	look	Look, mum.	
	nice	That's a nice T-shirt.	
	only	It's only five pounds.	

9	Sorry./I'm sorry.		
	have got	I've got (=I have got) twenty pence.	
	haven't (= have not) got	I haven't got a pound.	
	but	I've got ninety-nine pence, but I haven't got a pound.	

| **10** | plus | Seven plus six is thirteen. | |
| | minus ['maɪnəs] | Twenty minus six is fourteen. | |

11	can		
	help	Can I help you?	
	small		
	medium	Do you want your T-shirt small or medium?	
	take	Okay, I'll take it.	

12	paintbox		
	brush		
	get	Get a paintbox and a brush.	
	paint	Paint a butterfly on your T-shirt.	
	iron ['aɪən]	Iron the T-shirt.	
	put on	Put your T-shirt on.	
	make		
	parcel	Make a parcel.	
	open	Open the parcel.	
	(he/she/it) opens		
	there's (= there is)	There's a T-shirt in the parcel.	

UNIT 5

In an English classroom

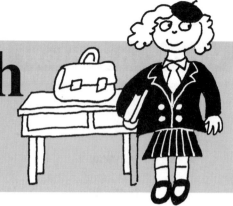

Revision

1

Grammar and vocabulary

How many short dialogues can you write?
Use these sentences:

How much is the T-shirt?

Hi, I'm Jenny. What's your name?

It's nine pounds sixty.

Let's have a party!

Do you like bananas?

Yes, thank you. We're fine.

No thank you. I hate sweets.

They're twenty pounds.

A party? Great idea.

Do you want a lolly?

Sandra.

No, I don't.

Simon and Peter, are you okay?

How much are the jeans?

2 *Read the text and colour in the clothes in the shop window.*

There is a yellow T-shirt with a blue and red butterfly on it, and a green T-shirt with a rainbow. The rainbow is red, blue, green, orange and yellow. On the pink jeans there is a green apple and a red lolly. On the blue jeans there is an orange apple and a pink lolly. There is a red star on the trainers and on the socks, but there is no star on the blouse. The trainers are blue and white, the socks are green and the blouse is white.

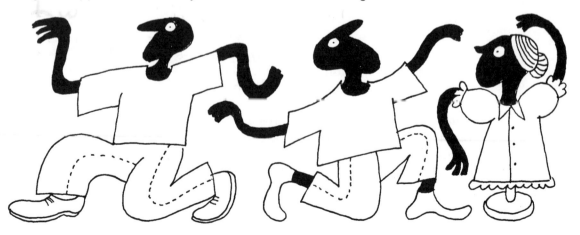

3 Using the words in the box, complete Colin's letter to his friend Peter.

Dear Peter,
    How _____ you?I ____ okay. I am in _____ 2b
We all _____ school uniforms: grey trousers,
a _____ grey pullover, a white shirt, a red
school _____ , a black blazer and black
_____ . I think my school uniform ___ nice.
Do you _____ a photo of my school?
            Yours,
                Colin.

wear

shoes

am

is

dark

are

tie

class

want

4 Write your opinion of these clothes. Use the words: **nice**, **okay**, **boring**, **ugly**.

school uniforms: **I think school uniforms look nice.** _____

pink jeans: _____

grey T-shirts: _____

white shoes: _____

blue and white trainers: _____

5 First write the correct numbers in the boxes below.
Then write the sentences under the pictures.

1	2	3	4
___	___	___	___

5	6	7	8
___	___	___	___

☐ Touch the floor.
☐ Shake your hair.
☐ Bend your knees.

☐ Jump.
☐ Put your right foot on your chair.

☐ Put your left foot on your chair.
☐ Stand up and clap your hands.
☐ Jump and turn around.

21

6 *Fill in what the teachers might say to the children in the following situations.*

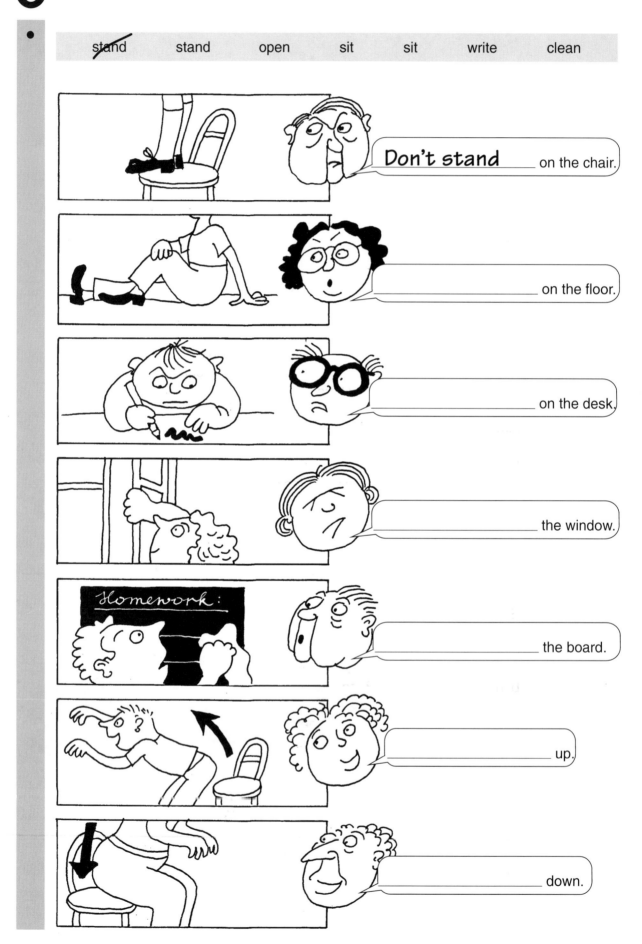

stand   stand   open   sit   sit   write   clean

Don't stand on the chair.

_____ on the floor.

_____ on the desk.

_____ the window.

_____ the board.

_____ up.

_____ down.

Words in context

*Write the words in
your language here:*

1

shut	Shut your book.	
listen to	Listen to the cassette.	
copy	Copy the sentences.	
clean	Clean the board, please.	
take out	Take out your books.	
homework		
hand out	Hand out the homework, please.	
quiet ['kwaɪət]	Be quiet, please.	
understand	Sorry, I don't understand.	
What's the homework?		

2

letter		
dear	Dear Peter,	
photo	Here is a photo of my school.	
wear [weə]	We all wear uniforms to school.	
dark	dark blue	
tie		
blazer		
think		
look		
boring	I think they look boring.	
Yours, Peter		

3

ugly	I think they look ugly.	
too	I think so too.	
I don't think so.		
I like wearing . . .		
So do I.		
I don't.		

4

clap	Clap your hands.	
bend	Bend your knees.	
foot		
left	your left foot	
right	your right hand	
put	Put your right foot on your chair.	
shake	Shake your hair.	

6

new	Is he new at our school?	
really	Is he really so cool?	
his eyes	His eyes are blue.	
always funny	What he says is always funny.	
write [raɪt]	Don't write on your hair.	

23

UNIT 6

Circus, circus

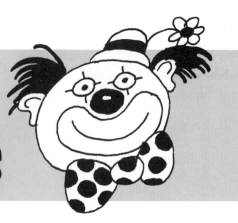

Revision

1

Vocabulary

Write the words in the lists.

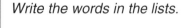

pink yellow chocolate hamburger
brown cassette recorder dark green board blouse
trousers hot dog
chewing gum floor door fruit gums desk
red T-shirt
toffee trainers ten coat ninety-nine
dress desk
chair blue overhead projector orange lolly jacket
two grey sixty sandwich three nineteen four
thirteen ice cream window tights

numbers	colours	in a classroom	sweets	snacks	clothes
ninety-nine	Yellow	door	fruitgums	Sandwich	dress
three	red	window	chocolate	hotdog	jacket
ten	Grange	chair	chewing gms	hamburg	coat
two	blue	desk	Icecream		
thirteen	brown	board			
sixty	pink				
nineteen	grey				
	darkgreen				

2 **Grammar**

How many questions can you make? Write them down.

| Do you like | How much are | How much is | Can I | Are you |

| Do you want | a toffee? | in Pam's class? | ice cream? |

| the sweater? | apples? | the socks? | alright? |

| help you? | open the window? | hungry? |

3 *Write the words.*

4 *Where are the pencil case, the biro, the schoolbag, the rubber and the pencil?*
Write sentences.

The pencil is behind the board.

_____

_____

_____

_____

5 *Write the sentences.*

is the Where mouse?

are snakes the Where?

to the the parrot apple Take.

caravan under frog is The the.

the behind snake caravan Is the?

Where is the mouse?

_____

_____

_____

_____

6 *Write the dialogue. First try to do this without checking in the Students' Book.*

■

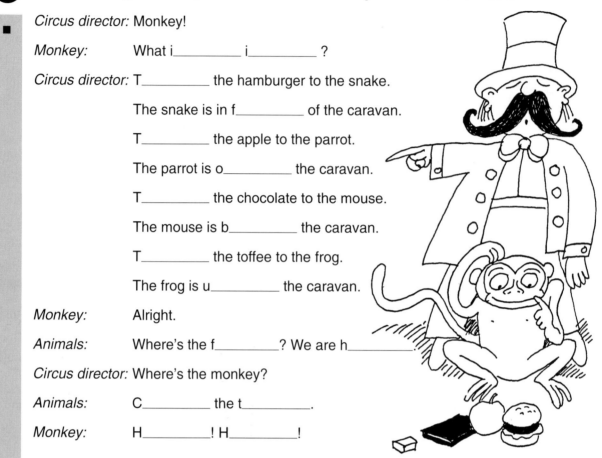

Circus director: Monkey!

Monkey: What i_____ i_____ ?

Circus director: T_____ the hamburger to the snake.

The snake is in f_____ of the caravan.

T_____ the apple to the parrot.

The parrot is o_____ the caravan.

T_____ the chocolate to the mouse.

The mouse is b_____ the caravan.

T_____ the toffee to the frog.

The frog is u_____ the caravan.

Monkey: Alright.

Animals: Where's the f_____? We are h_____.

Circus director: Where's the monkey?

Animals: C_____ the t_____.

Monkey: H_____! H_____!

7 *Read the text. Complete the picture of the circus director's caravan and colour it.*

•

The circus director's caravan is very funny. A blue snake is behind the curtain. A green snake is on the desk. A grey mouse is on the cupboard. A brown mouse is on the curtain. The frog is behind the pot plant. The monkey is in the wastepaper basket and the green parrot is on the chair. The blue parrot is in front of the desk. The floor is green. The curtains are orange and yellow. The cupboard is white and blue, the chair is orange and the wastepaper basket is pink. The desk is white.

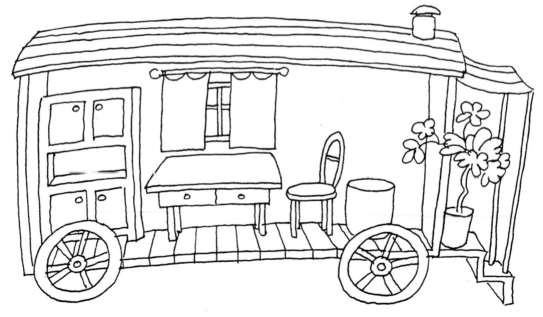

8 *Complete the dialogues.*

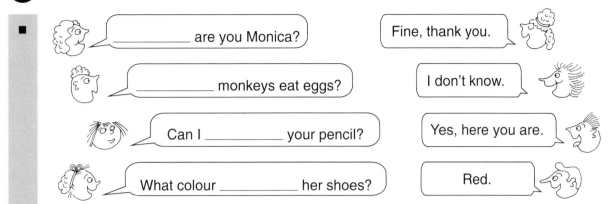

■ _____ are you Monica?

Fine, thank you.

_____ monkeys eat eggs?

I don't know.

Can I _____ your pencil?

Yes, here you are.

What colour _____ her shoes?

Red.

Wordfields

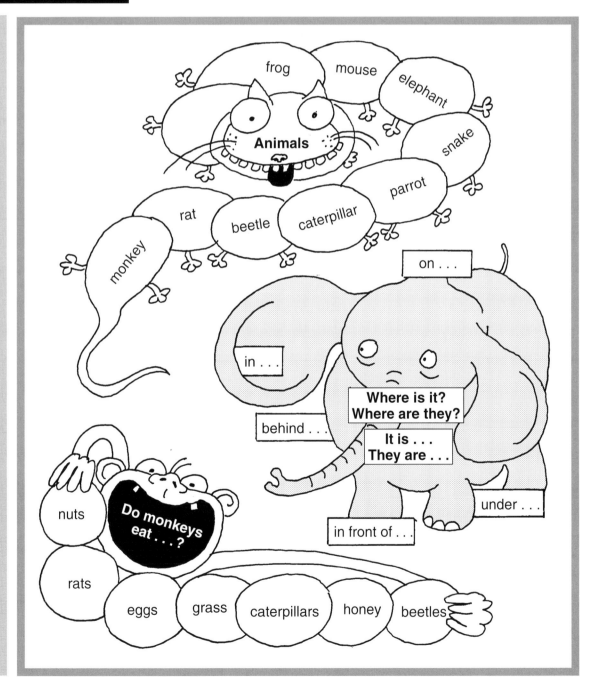

Words in context

*Write the words in
your language here:*

2 | where | Where is the frog?
| ear | It's in the elephant's ear.

3 | welcome
| the circus of the
talking animals
| circus director
| What is it?
| take to | Take the hamburger to the snake.
| caravan | The monkey is on the caravan.
| love | I love chocolate.
| wonderful | Toffees are wonderful.
| food | Where is the food?
| Catch the thief!

5 | again | Listen to the story again.

6 | hide | Hide the animals.
| letters | Write the letters in the picture.
| cupboard [ˈkʌbəd]
| wastepaper basket
| curtain
| pot plant

7 | Yes, it is.
| No, it isn't (= is not).

8 | eat | Do elephants eat eggs?
| don't (= do not) eat | They don't eat eggs.
| know | I don't know.

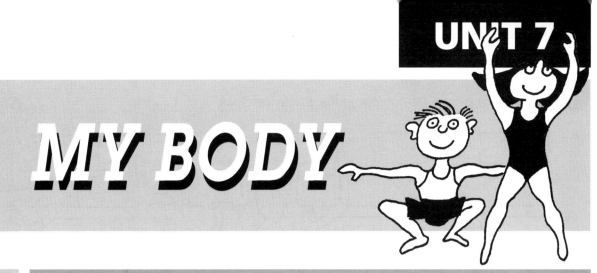

MY BODY

Revision

1 **Grammar**

Fill in the words from the box.

_____ you want a banana? No, I _____ like bananas.

Where are Fred and Simon? I think they _____ at John's party.

_____ you alright? No, I _____ very hungry.

Look. I _____ new jeans. They _____ super.

_____ I help you? No, thanks.

I like toffees, but I _____ like chewing gum.

are
are
am
don't
do
are
can
don't
have got

2 **Grammar**

Fill in: **a – an**

_____ new pot plant _____ egg for the snake _____ orange juice for Sandra

_____ nice ice cream _____ vanilla ice cream _____ sharpener

_____ rainbow _____ jacket _____ ugly shirt

_____ nice shirt _____ alphabet song _____ funny alphabet song

3 *Complete the questions.*

_____ much are the blue socks? – They're ten pounds fifty.

_____ is it? – Take the apple to the monkey.

_____ I help you? – Yes, please open the door for me.

_____ you like spearmint? – No, I hate it, but I like peppermint.

_____ the circus director in his caravan? – I don't think so.

_____ you hungry? – Yes, please give me a sandwich.

_____ do you want? – A lolly, please.

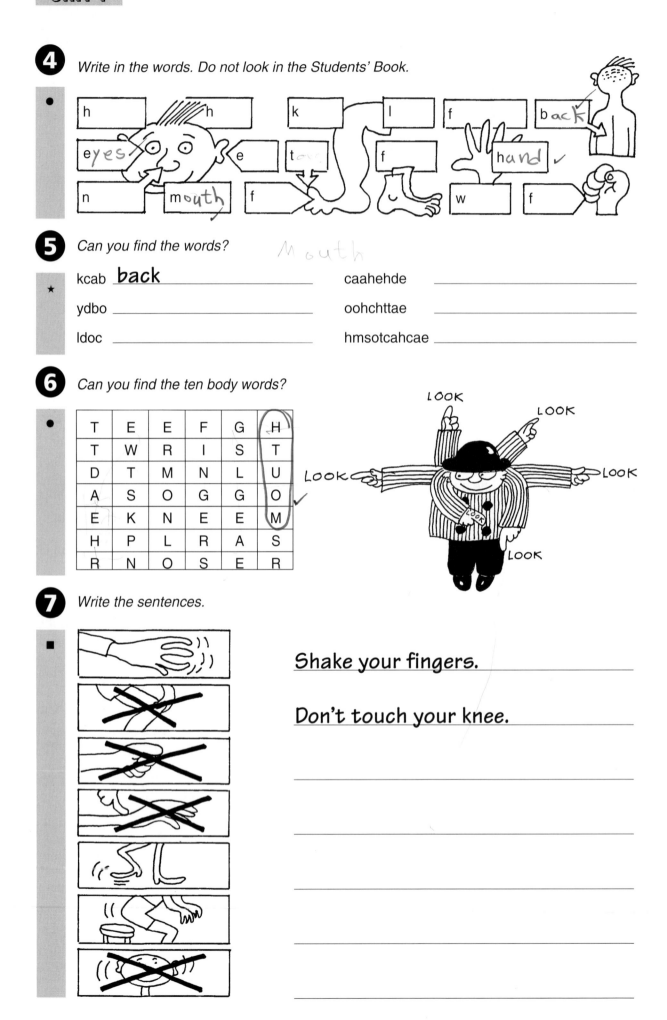

4 Write in the words. Do not look in the Students' Book.

5 Can you find the words?

kcab **back**

ydbo _____

ldoc _____

caahehde _____

oohchttae _____

hmsotcahcae _____

6 Can you find the ten body words?

T	E	E	F	G	H
T	W	R	I	S	T
D	T	M	N	L	U
A	S	O	G	G	O
E	K	N	E	E	M
H	P	L	R	A	S
R	N	O	S	E	R

LOOK LOOK LOOK LOOK LOOK

7 Write the sentences.

Shake your fingers. _____

Don't touch your knee. _____

_____

_____

_____

_____

_____

8 *How many mini dialogues can you write?*

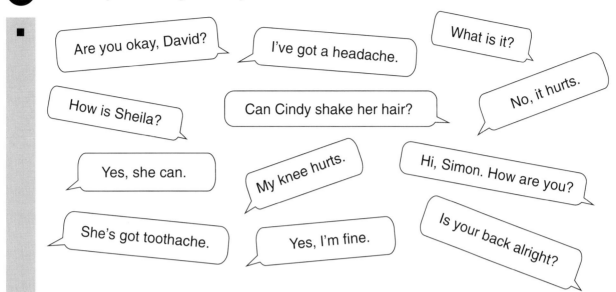

9 *Fill in:* **my – his – her**

Stanley, the lolly monster, is speaking about _____ mother and father:

"_____ mother's hair is green and _____ eyes are big and yellow. _____ ears are small, but _____ mouth is very big. _____ father's hair is red and _____ eyes are big and blue. It's funny, but _____ hair is blue and yellow, and _____ eyes are green and red. _____ father has got big legs, but_____ arms are very small. _____ mother has got small legs, but _____ arms are very big. It's funny, but _____ legs and_____ arms are big. I like _____ mother and _____ father. They are great."

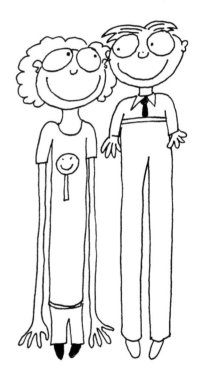

10 **Pronunciation**

★ *One word in each mouth is wrong. Which one is it? Underline it.*

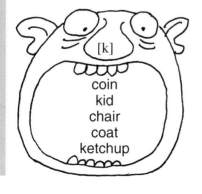

[k]
coin
kid
chair
coat
ketchup

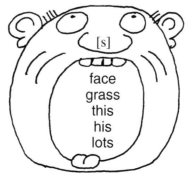

[s]
face
grass
this
his
lots

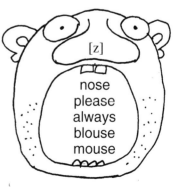

[z]
nose
please
always
blouse
mouse

Wordfield

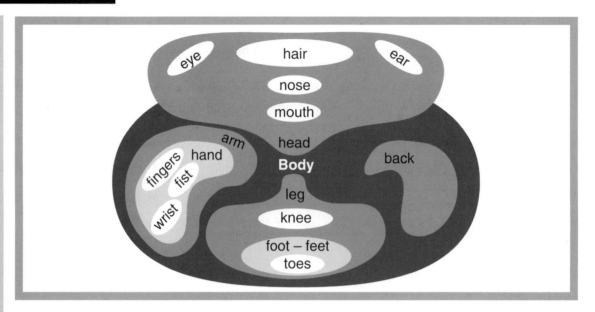

Words in context

Write the words in your language here:

3   close   Close your eyes.
       Take a seat.
       stamp   Stamp your feet.

4   hurt   My knee hurts.

5   today   How are you today?
       I'm not very well.
       a headache   I've got a headache.
       toothache   I've got toothache.
       stomachache   I've got stomachache.
       ['stʌməkeɪk]
       a cold   I've got a cold.

       can't (= cannot)   I can't come to the party.

6   lots of   The monster eats lots of lollies.
       he's (= he has) got   He's got a blue body.
       he hasn't   He hasn't got six feet.
       (= has not) got
       small   His ears are small.
       big   His mouth is big.

8   its   Look at the car. Its window
                         is open. Look at the snake.
                         Its mouth is very big.

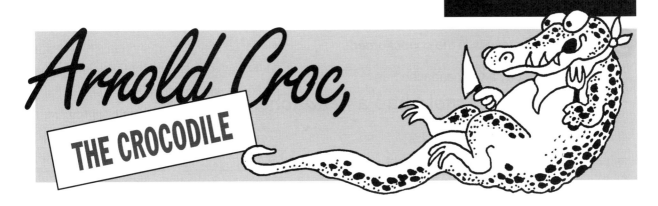

Arnold Croc,
THE CROCODILE

Revision

1

Grammar

Find Cynthia's school things. Write sentences.

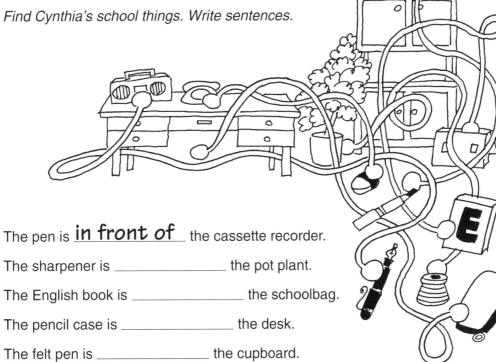

The pen is **in front of** the cassette recorder.

The sharpener is _____ the pot plant.

The English book is _____ the schoolbag.

The pencil case is _____ the desk.

The felt pen is _____ the cupboard.

The rubber is _____ the telephone.

2

★

Grammar

Fill in: **his – her – our – their**

Her friend Sylvia likes stories very much. (Sarah's)

Tom and I love spaghetti. It's _____ favourite food.

Where is _____ biro? (Rick's)

Give me _____ exercise book, please. (Sue's)

_____ friend Susie is in my class. (Joanne's)

_____ books are under the desk. (Peter's and Ann's)

33

3 *Write the sentences in the correct order.*

• Arnold Tuesday a On headache has

On Tuesday Arnold has a headache.

cold Arnold On a has Monday.

_____

knee On Arnold's Wednesday hurts.

_____

On the to Sunday goes banana tree Arnold.

_____

On on the back Saturday jumps frog Arnold's.

_____

On and Arnold Friday toothache has Thursday.

_____

4 *Cross out the ten words that do not belong to the story.*
Write the words down and write the words that are correct.

■ elephant → crocodile

Bad luck for Arnold

Arnold Croc, the elephant, eats parrots, ducks and cats. He doesn't like apples, bananas or oranges. He eats monkeys, snakes and frogs. He doesn't like chocolate, fruit gums or English books.
Arnold Croc makes a plan for the week. He writes a song.
Arnold Croc, the crocodile, looks at the list and smiles.
Monday is a bad day for Arnold. He has a cold. No trainers for Arnold.

On Tuesday Arnold has a headache. No duck for Arnold.
On Wednesday Arnold's knee hurts. No homework for Arnold.
On Thursday and Friday Arnold has toothache. No monkey and no snake for Arnold.
On Saturday the mouse jumps on Arnold's nose. "Where's the frog?" Arnold says. He is very ugly. And he is very, very pink.
On Sunday Arnold goes to the circus. He eats and eats and eats. Then he has stomachache. Bad luck for Arnold.

5 *Fill in the correct plural forms.*

■

five _____

three _____

two _____

three _____

some _____

five _____

lots of good _____

6 *Fill in:* **like – likes**

★ I ___like___ bananas and apples.

Arnold Croc _____ snakes, parrots and monkeys.

Rick, Tina and Pam _____ Sarah's party.

The circus director _____ his animals.

Nick Sellers _____ school uniforms.

I _____ wearing jeans and sweaters.

John _____ wearing his white and blue trainers to school.

7 *Fill in:* **don't – doesn't**

● I ___don't___ think school uniforms are ugly.

Arnold _____ eat oranges and he _____ like apples.

Sarah's mother _____ like fruit gums.

Jim and Sandra _____ eat sweets.

Jenny _____ go to my class, she goes to class 1 b.

Thomas and I _____ like pink.

Frank likes bananas, but he _____ like apples.

I like juice, but I _____ like coffee.

Nora likes reading, but she _____ like comics.

8 *Write sentences.*

■ John /☺/ sweets

John likes sweets. _____

The monkey /☺/ ice cream and chocolate

_____

The crocodile /☺/ frogs

_____

Rita /☹/ school uniforms

_____

☞ **p. t. o. (please turn over)**

Peter / 😐 / black T-shirts

_____

Oliver / 🙂 / strawberry ice cream

_____

Sheila / 🙁 / chocolate ice cream

_____

9 _Read this text and complete the picture._

It is Sunday. Arnold is under the big banana tree. He has stomachache.
He has a big pencil in his hand.

And here is his list:

Food for Monday: orange juice
Food for Tuesday: orange juice
Food for Wednesday: orange juice
Food for Thursday: orange juice
Food for Friday: an apple
Food for Saturday: an apple and a carrot
Food for Sunday: an orange

There are lots of animals with Arnold.
The parrot is in the tree.
The duck is in front of Arnold.
The cat is on Arnold's back and the monkey is behind Arnold.
"We're sorry for Arnold," they all say and smile.

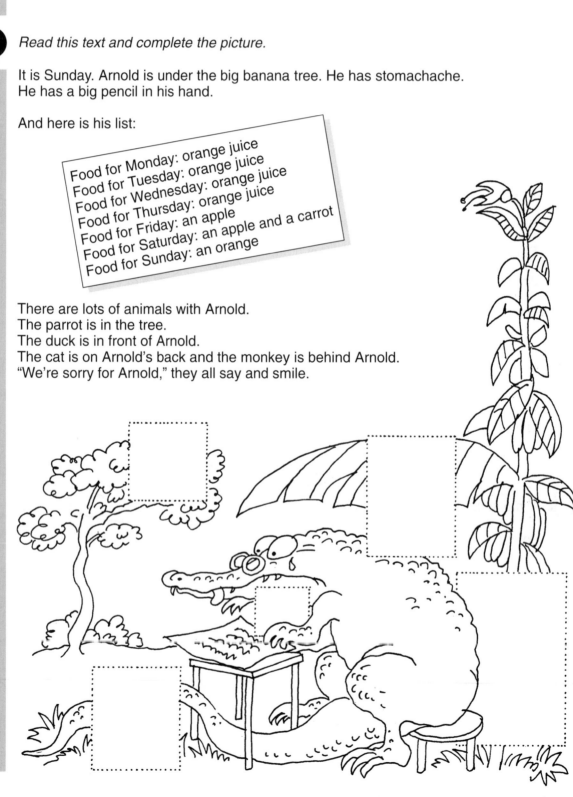

Wordfield

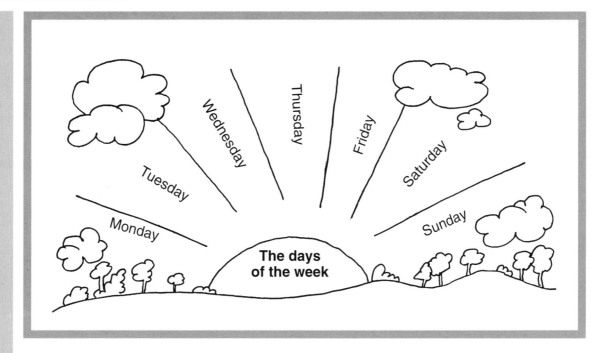

The days of the week

Monday · Tuesday · Wednesday · Thursday · Friday · Saturday · Sunday

Words in context

Write the words in your language here:

1	dentist	Go to the dentist.	
3	crocodile		
	doesn't (= does not) like	Arnold doesn't like popcorn.	
	plan	Arnold makes a plan for the week.	
	list	He writes a list.	
	look at	Arnold looks at the list.	
	smile	He smiles.	
	bad	Monday is a bad day for Arnold.	
	angry	Arnold is very angry.	
	tree	Arnold goes to the banana tree.	
	bad luck	This is bad luck for Arnold.	
6	bed	He is in bed.	

UNIT 9

What's the time?

Revision

1 Vocabulary

Write down the words.

nineteen plus seventeen = <u>thirty-six</u>

eighty-three plus thirteen = _____

twenty-nine plus forty-three = _____

eighty-seven plus eleven = _____

seventy-three minus thirty-seven = _____

a hundred minus eighty-one = _____

twenty-four plus forty-three = _____

sixty-seven minus twenty-four = _____

ninety-three minus sixteen = _____

eighteen plus fifty-seven = _____

2 Grammar and vocabulary

What's wrong with them? Write sentences.

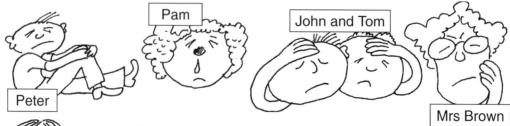

Pam

John and Tom

Mrs Brown

Peter

<u>Peter's knee hurts.</u>

_____

_____

_____

Nancy

_____

38

3 **Grammar**

Fill in: **like – likes – don't like – doesn't like**

Arnold ☹ _**doesn't like**_ bananas,

he ☺ _____ ducks and cats.

I ☺ _____ sweets. I ☹ _____ milk.

Five boys in my class ☺ _____ ice cream.

Phil and Mark ☹ _____ hot dogs.

We ☺ _____ Disneyland.

Nancy ☺ _____ popcorn.

4 *Colour the clocks and watches.*

green: ten to eight
pink: five to one
blue: half past one
red: twenty-five past three
orange: half past nine
white: ten to two
yellow: twenty past eight
orange and blue: quarter to nine
blue and white: twenty to five
brown: quarter past twelve
blue and red: twenty-five to four

5 *Mark the sentences true (T) or false (F).*

Brian's day

☐ Brian gets up at half past seven.

☐ He has breakfast at quarter to eight.

☐ He goes to school at twenty-five past eight.

☐ School starts at ten to nine.

☐ School ends at half past four.

☐ He gets home at five to five.

☐ He goes to bed at nine o'clock.

6 *Fill in the correct forms of the verbs in the box.*

★

Tom __*gets up*__ at half past seven.

I always _____ breakfast at seven o'clock.

Mary is from London. School _____ at nine o'clock and

_____ at four o'clock.

For Pierre and Françoise from Paris, school _____ at nine o'clock

and _____ at five o'clock.

I _____ to school at quarter past seven.

For me school _____ at quarter to eight.

For Mike and Pam school _____ at half past three.

Then they _____ TV or _____ with friends.

play

go

start

start

have

~~get up~~

end

start

end

watch

end

7 *Complete the following sentences.*

•

I get up at _____. I get home at _____.

I have breakfast at _____. Then I _____.

I go to school at _____. I go to bed at _____.

8 *Complete the following poem. Fill in the rhyme words from the box.*

■

| hair | fine | shoe | four | fine | ~~late~~ | pen | TV |

School starts at ten to eight,

but I am always ___*late*___.

English starts at ten to nine,

and that is really _____.

Spanish starts at twenty to ten,

and I haven't got my _____.

It's not on my desk, or under my chair.

Oh, here it is, in Susan's _____.

School ends at five past two,

and I haven't got my _____.

Oh, here it is, behind the door.

I'm late again, it's half past _____.

At five o'clock I have my tea.

At ten to six I watch _____.

I go to bed at nine,

and I don't think that's _____.

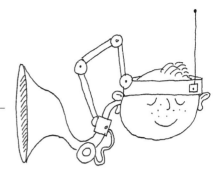

9 Pronunciation

Which one sounds different?

big sit fist five listen ___five___

angry alright animal apple alphabet _____

arm car game class half past _____

fit seat feet sweet please _____

Wordfields

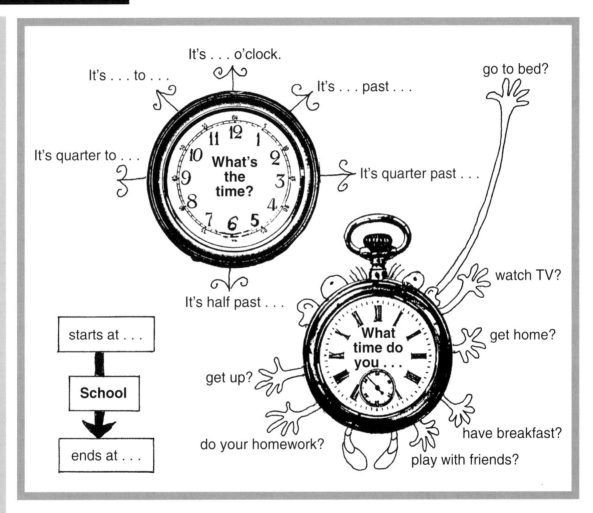

It's . . . o'clock.

It's . . . to . . .

It's . . . past . . .

go to bed?

It's quarter to . . .

What's the time?

It's quarter past . . .

It's half past . . .

starts at . . .

↓

School

↓

ends at . . .

get up?

do your homework?

What time do you . . .

watch TV?

get home?

have breakfast?

play with friends?

Words in context

Write the words in your language here:

2	watch	That's a nice watch.
7	hour [aʊə]	

UNIT 10

That's me!

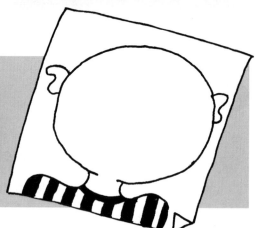

Revision

1

Grammar

Fill in the missing words.

Sarah likes _____ school uniform. It is red and blue.

Paul can't touch _____ toes.

I like hamburgers. _____ mother hates them.

Peter and Claire don't like _____ teacher.

We don't like _____ classroom. It is very cold.

"Open _____ books at page 27, please."

"Please, Mrs Thompson, can you help me with _____ homework?"

"Jane, is this _____ pen?" "No, I think it's Mike's."

"Is this Anna's bike?" "No, _____ bike is green."

Can a snake touch _____ nose?

| my |
| my |
| your |
| his |
| her |
| its |
| our |
| their |
| your |
| her |

2

Vocabulary

Find words for the letters.

A _is for apple_ .   J _____ .   S _____ .

B _is for bird_ .   K _____ .   T _____ .

C _is for cat_ .   L _____ .   U _____ .

D _____ .   M _____ .   V _____ .

E _____ .   N _____ .   W _____ .

F _____ .   O _____ .   X _is for Xmas_
                                        (= Christmas) .

G _____ .   P _____ .

H _____ .   Q _____ .   Y _____ .

I _____ .   R _____ .   Z _is for zoo_ .

3 Grammar and vocabulary

What's the time in Moscow, San Francisco and Sydney?
Write in the correct times.

MOSCOW	SAN FRANCISCO	SYDNEY
13.00	2.00	20.00
It's one pm in Moscow.	It's two am in San Francisco.	It's eight pm in Sydney.
7.00		
It's seven am in Moscow.		
	5.30	
	It's five thirty am in San Francisco.	
		13.15
		It's one fifteen pm in Sydney.
23.45		
It's eleven forty-five pm in Moscow.		
	24.00	
	It's midnight in San Francisco.	

4 *Write the words.*

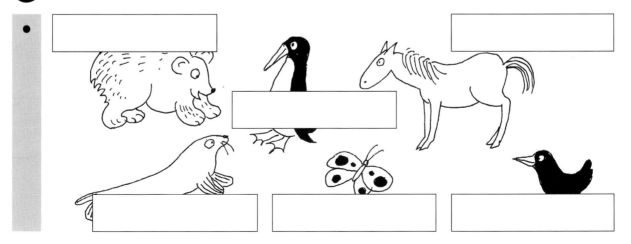

5 *Write sentences.*

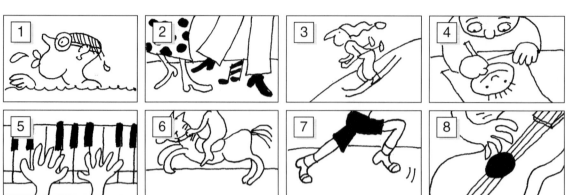

Henry (8 + 5 –) "_I'm good at playing the guitar, but I'm_
not very good at playing the piano.   "

Mary (1 + 3 +) "_I'm good at swimming and I'm good_
at skiing.   "

John (1 + 7 –) "_____

_____ "

Susan (5 + 6 +) "_____

_____ "

David (2 – 8 –) "_____

_____ "

Jenny (1 + 8 +) "_____

_____ "

Chris (3 + 4 +) "_____

_____ "

Janet (4 – 5 +) "_____

_____ "

Peter (1 + 7 –) "_____

_____ "

Carol (3 – 6 +) "_____

_____ "

Tom (6 + 8 +) "_____

_____ "

Angela (4 – 7 –) "_____

_____ "

Wordfield

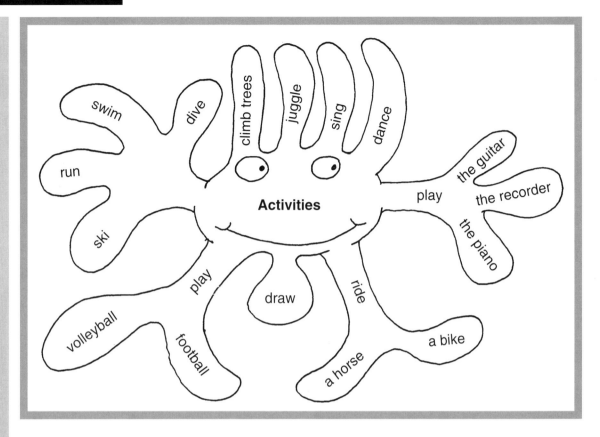

Words in context

*Write the words in
your language here:*

2	truth	Can you tell the truth?	
3	good at	Are you good at drawing?	
6	penguin	Percy, the penguin, has two friends.	
	bear		
	blackbird	The blackbird is Percy's friend.	
	laugh	The bear laughs and climbs a tree.	
	nothing	That's nothing.	
	sad	Percy is sad.	
	go away	He goes away.	
	juggle	Can you juggle?	
	please		
	teach	Please, teach me to juggle.	
	go back	Percy goes back to his friends.	
	at this moment		
	baby bird		
	fall into	A baby bird falls into the water.	
	shout	They all shout, "Help, help!"	

UNIT 11

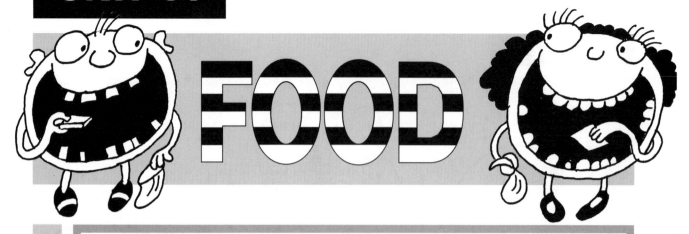

FOOD

Revision

1 **Vocabulary**

Sort out the words and write them down in three lists.

orange juice
cabbage
coke
tomato
toffee
milk shake
chocolate
fruit gum
spinach
ice cream
water
apple juice
carrot
bread beans
cheese
lolly
coffee
egg

Food

Things to drink

Sweet things

2 **Grammar**

What they like

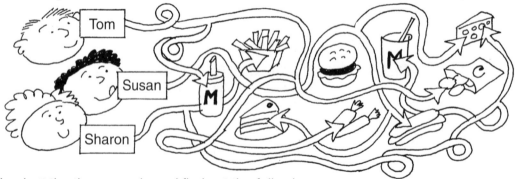

Tom

Susan

Sharon

Look at the three people and find out the following:

What does Tom like? _____

What does Sharon like? _____

What does Susan like? _____

3 Food bingo

Choose five things on the bingo card. Write the words on a piece of paper. When your teacher reads out the words you have got, cross them out on the bingo card (use a pencil). Call out "Bingo!" when you have all five.

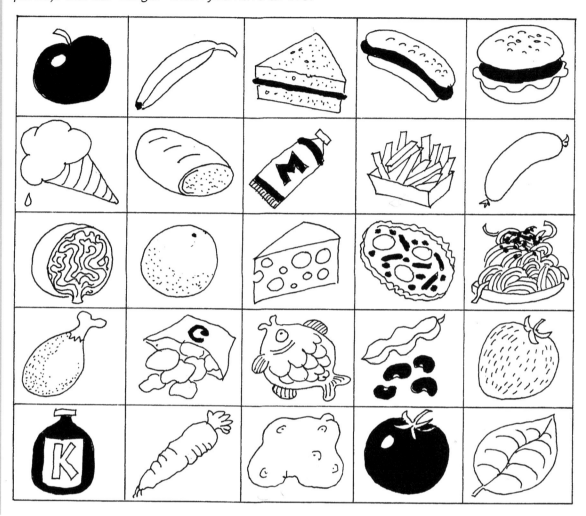

4 *What do you like? And what don't you like? Make notes.*

	Fast food	Vegetables	Drinks	Sweets
I like	chips	carrot	fizzy drinks	Ice cream
I don't like		onions	tea	

Now write it down.

Fast food: I like _____ ,

　　　　　　 but I don't like _____ .

Vegetables: I like _____ ,

　　　　　　 but I don't like _____ .

Drinks: I like _____ ,

　　　　　　 but I don't like _____ .

Sweets: I like _____ ,

　　　　　　 but I don't like _____ .

5 **Pronunciation**

★ *Put the words in two lists.*

their
thank
that
think
thief
thirteen
then
thirty
Thursday
the
there
three
through
they
mother
father

[θ] thing　　　　　　　　[ð] this

_____ _____　　_____ _____

_____ _____　　_____ _____

_____ _____　　_____ _____

_____ _____　　_____ _____

6 *Find the correct order and write down the sentences.*

■ hamburgers Does like Peter ?   _____

doesn't he No, .   _____

Peter like What does ?   _____

and chicken likes chips He   _____

he vegetables like Does ?   _____

does he Yes, .   _____

favourite his vegetable What is ?   _____

Wordfields

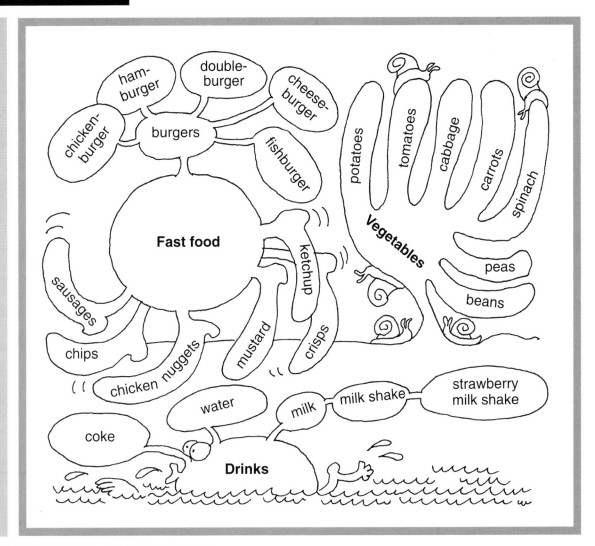

Words in context

Write the words in your language here:

2	menu ['menjʊ]	Can I have the menu, please?	
	large	I want a small/medium/large milk shake, please.	
	Anything else?		
3	restaurant	Let's go to the fast-food restaurant.	
	Next, please.		
4	cheese	I don't like cheese.	
5	favourite	Carrots are my favourite vegetable.	
	what	What vegetable do you hate?	

collecting things

Revision

1 Grammar

Fill in:

my	*Frank and Sue:* In _____ group, four girls collect postcards.
my	*Carol:* Maria, can I look at _____ comics?
my	*Sharon:* Hey, Sandy. Give me back _____ coins.
your	*Teacher:* Open _____ books at page 26.
your	*Tom and Tina:* All _____ phonecards are from England.
our	*Vanessa:* I love The Swampers. I've got all _____ autographs.
our	*Cathy:* I can't find _____ books. Chris, can you help me?
their	
their	*Teacher:* The girls in _____ class all put stickers on _____ schoolbags.

2 Grammar and vocabulary

Fill in numbers 1 to 10.

1	How much is			the mouse? – Under the chair.
2	What's			you? – Fine, thank you.
3	What flavour			is it? – Ten past three.
4	Where's			is it? – Peppermint.
5	What colour is			the jeans? – £35.
6	Do you want			your mountain bike? – Green.
7	How are			your telephone number? – 3-0-7-7-5-6.
8	What colour are		*1*	the sweater? – It's £62.
9	What time			a sweet, Cathy? – No, thank you.
10	How much are			her trainers? – White and red.

3 *Colour the flags and then write the names of the countries below them.*

● green

_____ _____ _____ _____

_____ _____ _____ _____

4 *Write down the two dialogues in the correct order.*

●
- [ ] Only six.
- [ ] Yes. Do you collect phonecards too?
- [1] What do you collect?
- [ ] How many have you got?
- [ ] Yes, I do.
- [ ] A hundred and twenty.
- [ ] How many phonecards have you got?
- [ ] Comics.
- [ ] Wow. That's a lot.
- [1] Can I have a look at your phonecards, Susan?

5 *Fill in the words from the box.*

●
got
~~me~~
is
are
lot
are
got
them
you
me

Claire: Can you give __me__ some stamps?

Ralph: How many do _____ want?

Claire: How many have you _____ ?

Ralph: I've _____ thirty.

Claire: Can you give _____ ten?

Ralph: Ten? That's a _____ . What can you give me for _____?

Claire: Ten badges. _____ that okay?

Ralph: Yes. Here _____ the stamps.

Claire: Here _____ the badges.

6 *Put the text into the correct order.*

★

[ ] Then George sees a woman with a very old cat under the tree. "I'm so hungry," says the old woman. So George swaps his pig for the very old cat. Then he walks home.

[1] George works for a farmer. The farmer gives him a horse. George is happy and gets on his horse to ride home.

[ ] So they swap animals. The old man is very happy and rides away on the horse.

[ ] George is happy. Now he can buy a lot of food for his old cat.

[ ] The old man looks very tired and is walking very slowly. "Take my horse and give me your pig," says George.

[ ] Now he is tired and hungry. "Miaow," says the cat. "Poor thing. You are hungry." So George goes out to catch a mouse for the hungry old cat. The cat goes with George.

[ ] He pulls and pulls. It's a bag. He opens it. "What's that?" It is full of gold coins.

[ ] The sun is hot and he stops under a tree. Suddenly he sees an old man with a pig.

[ ] It stops in front of a mouse hole. George puts in his hand to catch a mouse for the cat. "But what's that?" George feels something hard.

7 *Fill in the missing words and then number the correct answers.*

■

1	**What** do you collect?	( ) 39.
2	_____ you give me ten stamps?	( ) Yes, I do.
3	_____ you got a British phonecard?	( ) No, she collects stickers.
4	_____ many comics have you got?	( ) Yes, of course. Do you like comics?
5	_____ you collect stickers too, David?	( ) No, only two.
6	_____ I have a look at your comics?	(7) Stickers.
7	_____ Carol collect stamps too?	( ) No, I haven't.

8 *Can you find seven words for things you can collect?*

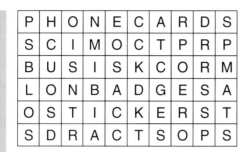

P	H	O	N	E	C	A	R	D	S
S	C	I	M	O	C	T	P	R	P
B	U	S	I	S	K	C	O	R	M
L	O	N	B	A	D	G	E	S	A
O	S	T	I	C	K	E	R	S	T
S	D	R	A	C	T	S	O	P	S

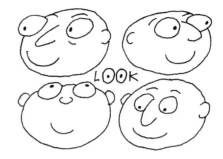

9 **Pronunciation**

One word in each monster is wrong. Which one is it? Underline it.

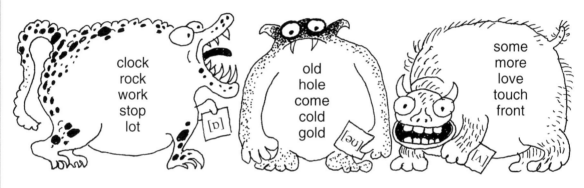

clock
rock
work
stop
lot

[ɒ]

old
hole
come
cold
gold

[əʊ]

some
more
love
touch
front

[ʌ]

Wordfields

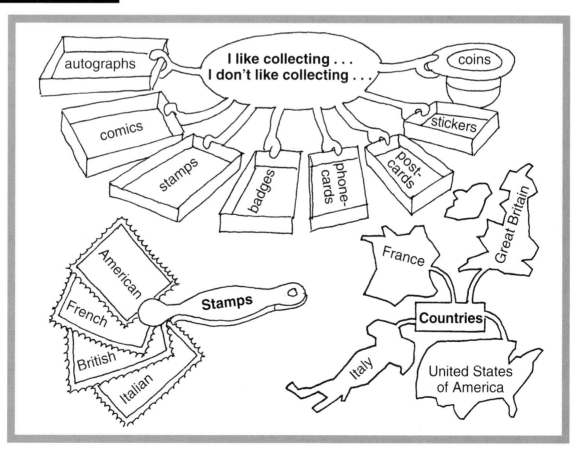

I like collecting . . .
I don't like collecting . . .

autographs   coins

comics   stickers

stamps   badges   phone-cards   post-cards

Stamps
American
French
British
Italian

Countries
France
Great Britain
Italy
United States of America

Words in context

*Write the words in
your language here:*

2 collect — What do you collect?
how many — How many stickers have you got?
about — about sixty

4 Yes, of course.
a lot of/lots of — I've got a lot of/lots of coins.
too — Do you collect badges too?
footballer — I collect autographs of footballers.
aunt — I have an aunt in America.
send — She sends me lots of stamps.

7 dad — My dad collects coins.
envelope — Can I have this envelope with the American stamp on it?
scissors ['sizəz] — Get some scissors.
fill — Fill a glass with water.
wait — Wait for twenty minutes.
hairdryer
sail out — The stamp sails out of the window.
try — Try to catch it.

9 generous ['dʒenərəs] — He is very generous.
work — George works for a farmer.
him — The farmer gives him a horse.
get on — George gets on his horse.
sun — The sun is hot.
stop — Stop this!
sofa — It's under the sofa.
pig — George swapped his pig.
suddenly — Suddenly George sees an old man.
tired — You look tired.
ride away — The old man rides away on the horse.
Poor thing!
mouse hole — The cat stops in front of the mouse hole.
feel
hard — George feels something hard.
pull — He pulls and pulls.
bag — The bag is full of gold coins.
buy — With the gold coins, George can buy a lot of food.

10 right
wrong

The swapping game

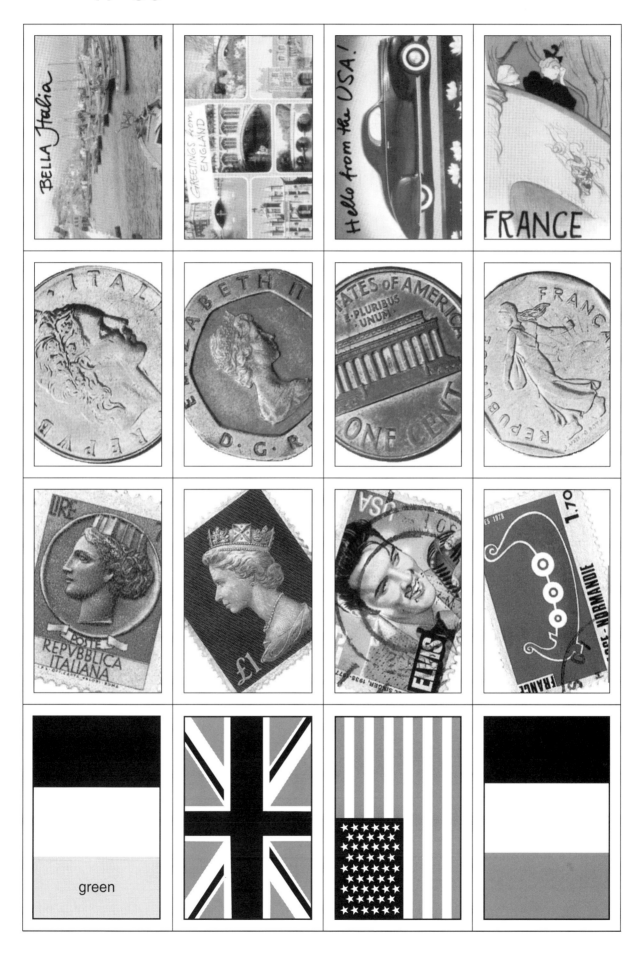

ROOMS

FOR RENT

Revision

1 **Vocabulary**

Do you know the English words? Write them down.

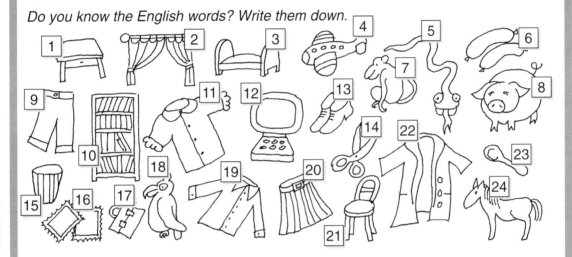

2 **Grammar and vocabulary**

Mark the words in the box and write down sentences.

* means: I am good at it.

+ means: I like it.

– means: I do not like it.

o means: I am not good at it.

⊛	climbing	⊕	hamburgers
○	English	○	swimming
○	dancing	○	football
○	mustard	○	juggling
○	volleyball	○	horse riding
○	milk	○	spinach
○	swapping	○	shopping
○	rock 'n' roll	○	watching TV
○	playing the piano		

Examples:

I am *good* at climbing.
I like hamburgers.

3 *Write down the names of the rooms.*

■ htcenik _____ reobodm _____

tomabhor _____ vnglii mroo _____

4 *Write down what you think the people are doing.*

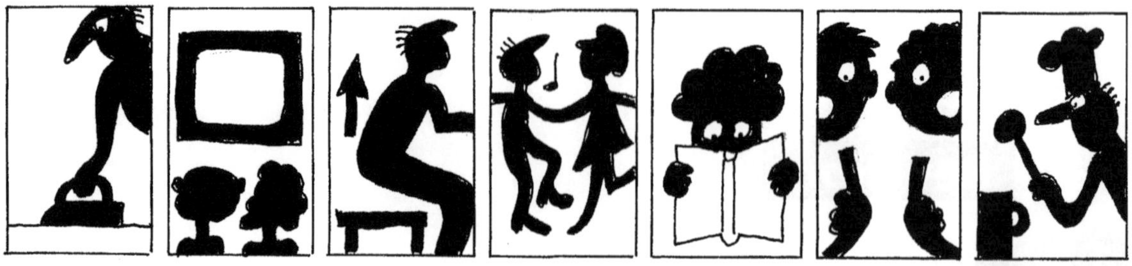

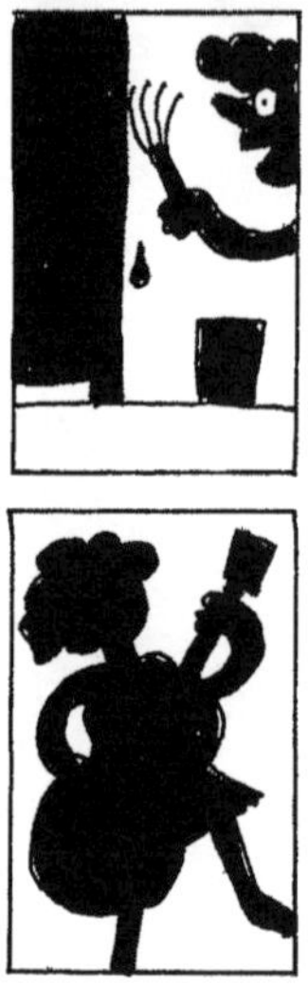

■

I think the man is ironing a shirt.

_____

_____

_____

_____

_____

_____

_____

_____

5 *Complete the dialogues.*

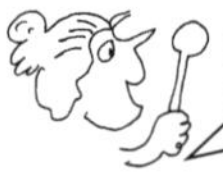

■ Can you help me with the cooking?

Oh Mum, I'm watching a video.

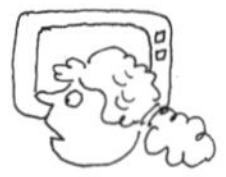

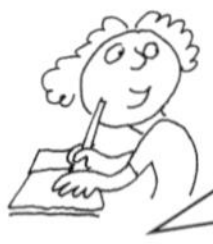

_____

Not now, I'm reading my book.

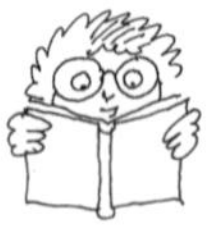

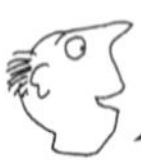

David, time to go to bed.

_____

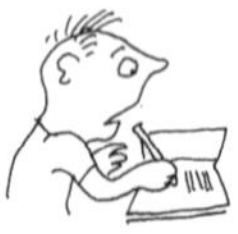

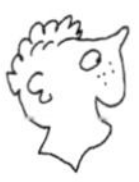

Can you help me, James?

_____

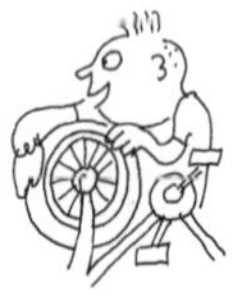

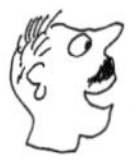

Can you help me in the garden, Sue?

_____

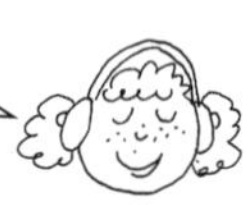

6 *Join the letters. Listen to your teacher.*

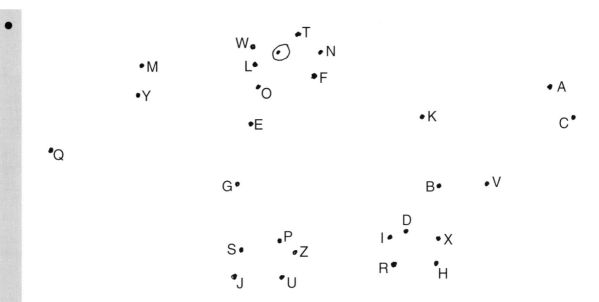

7 *Spot the difference. Write down the sentences. Start like this:*

■ In picture A there are three pot plants,
in picture B there are two.

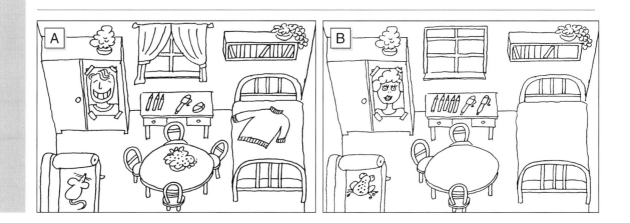

8 Spelling bingo

Choose five words on the bingo card. Write the words on a piece of paper.
When your teacher spells the words you have got, cross them out on the bingo card
(use a pencil). Call out "Bingo!" when you have all five.

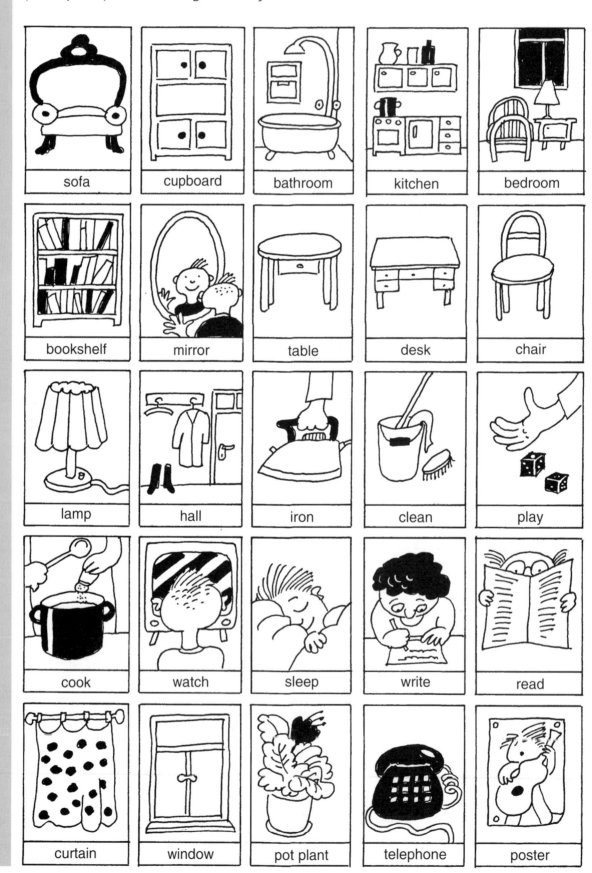

sofa	cupboard	bathroom	kitchen	bedroom
bookshelf	mirror	table	desk	chair
lamp	hall	iron	clean	play
cook	watch	sleep	write	read
curtain	window	pot plant	telephone	poster

Wordfields

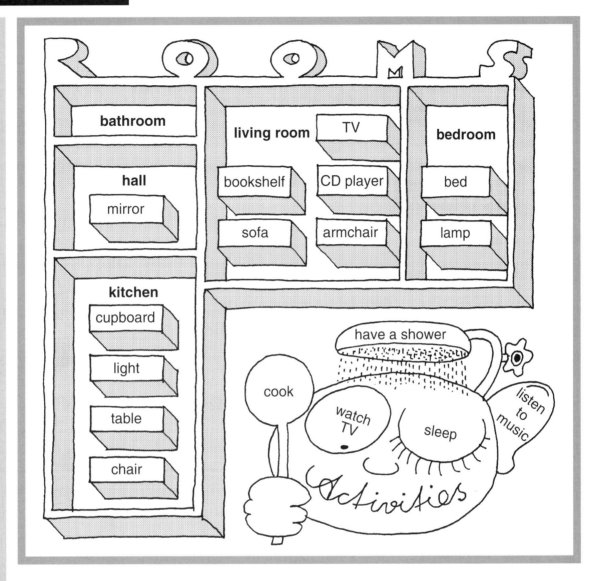

ROOMS

bathroom

hall
mirror

kitchen
cupboard
light
table
chair

living room | TV
bookshelf | CD player
sofa | armchair

bedroom
bed
lamp

have a shower
cook
watch TV
sleep
listen to music
activities

Words in context

Write the words in your language here:

| 3 | noise | |
| | who | Who is making that noise? |

| 4 | poster | In Carol's room there is a poster of an elephant. |

| 6 | flat | John is in his flat. |

| 9 | film | Can I watch this film on TV? |
| | go shopping | Can you go shopping for me, please? |

Happy Birthday

Revision

1

Grammar

Write the dialogues.

Can you come to my house?

No, I'm sorry. **I'm doing my homework.**

Do you want to play football?

No, I'm sorry. I_____

_____

Do you want to go shopping?

No, _____

_____

Do you want to come for a bike ride?

No, _____

_____

Do you want to go to a fast-food restaurant?

No, _____

_____

Do you want to go swimming?

No, _____

_____

2 Vocabulary

Write the words in three lists.

sofa   ~~postcards~~   draw   table   dance   **SKI**

stamps   **light**   stickers   *paint*   *comics*   autographs   chair

bookshelf   CD player   armchair

dive   **coins**   swim   TV   play   **run**

badges

Things to collect:	Activities:	In the living room:
postcards		

3 Write the ordinals of the numbers in words.

4	the fourth	40		72	
15		48		80	
20		59		90	
26		61		94	
37		68		100	

4 *Write the birthdays. Check with your calendar.*

Claire: 3/12/19 . . <u>**Claire's birthday is on December 3rd.**</u>
<u>**It's on a**_____**day this year.**</u>
(Fill in the day.)

Christopher 2/6/19 . . _____

_____

Cathy 14/7/19 . . _____

_____

Rick 23/1/19 . . _____

_____

Sarah 18/2/19 . . _____

_____

Jim 6/3/19 . . _____

_____

Tina 17/5/19 . . _____

_____

5 *Put the sentences into the correct order. Write numbers in the boxes.*

Maggie's birthday present

☐ There's a plastic bowl, a rubber ball and a big brown brush!
☐ Then they all go out into the garden.
☐ First she opens the presents from her friends.
☐ It is Maggie's present from her brothers and her mother.
☐ There in a basket is a beautiful little dog.
☐ They eat lots of the birthday cake, and then Maggie opens her presents.
☐ The bowl, the brush and the ball are really for the dog.
1 It is Maggie's eleventh birthday.
☐ She gets home from school at five o'clock and has a party with her family and friends.
☐ Then she opens the presents from her brothers and her mother.
☐ There's a book, a biro and a music cassette. Maggie is very happy.
☐ In the morning she opens her birthday cards and then she goes to school.

Wordfields

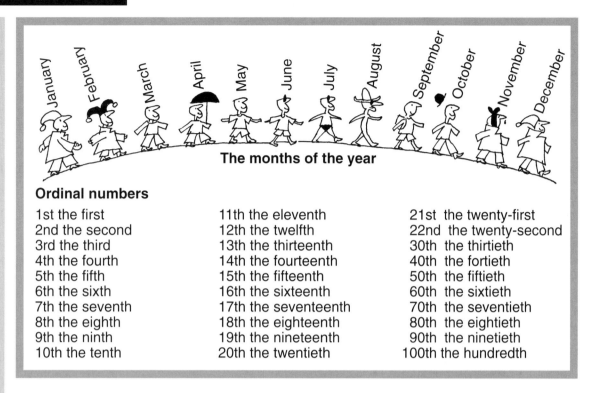

The months of the year

January February March April May June July August September October November December

Ordinal numbers

1st the first	11th the eleventh	21st the twenty-first
2nd the second	12th the twelfth	22nd the twenty-second
3rd the third	13th the thirteenth	30th the thirtieth
4th the fourth	14th the fourteenth	40th the fortieth
5th the fifth	15th the fifteenth	50th the fiftieth
6th the sixth	16th the sixteenth	60th the sixtieth
7th the seventh	17th the seventeenth	70th the seventieth
8th the eighth	18th the eighteenth	80th the eightieth
9th the ninth	19th the nineteenth	90th the ninetieth
10th the tenth	20th the twentieth	100th the hundredth

Words in context

*Write the words in
your language here:*

2
birthday	
when	When is Judith's birthday?
what day	What day is it this year?

3
present	Here is your birthday present.
candle	
birthday cake	Put the candles on the birthday cake.
plastic bowl [bəʊl]	
birthday card	In the morning Maggie opens her birthday cards.
family	She has three cards from her family.
schoolfriend	Maggie has a party with her schoolfriends.
brother	Her brother is ten years old.
music cassette	Do you like this music cassette?
rubber ball	Maggie's brother gives her a rubber ball.
Thank you very much.	
find	Maggie opens her mother's present and finds a brush.
little	In the basket there is a little dog for Maggie.
kiss	Maggie kisses the dog.

Breakfast

Revision

1 **Grammar and vocabulary**

Fill in the correct plural forms.

five stamps _____

_____ _____

_____ _____

_____ _____

_____ _____

_____

2 **Grammar and vocabulary**

Write the sentences.

you / like / swimming / David ? / Do

Do you like swimming, David? _____

Jane / goes / school / 8.30 . / at / to

_____

In the morning / all her / Maggie / opens / birthday cards .

_____

Munchie / like / spinach? / Does – No / he / not . / does

_____

Munchie and Crunchie / Do / eat / frogs? – No / do / they / not .

_____

do / What / you / collect? – I / not / collect / things . / do

_____

How many / you / got /stamps / have ?

_____

Generous George / gets / on / horse / and / rides / home . / his

_____

the cat / catch / Does / the mouse? – No / he / not . / does

_____

of / There / lot / books / on the bookshelf . / are / a

_____

3 *Find all the food words.*

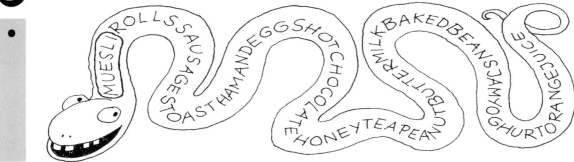

4 *The letters of these words are jumbled. Write them out correctly.*

★

toguyrh	**yoghurt**	slorl	
rtbetu		focefe	
skraocnlfe		nhyeo	
tlehooacc		snabe	

5 *Fill in:* **a – an – some**.

Would you like _____ **an** _____ egg?

I'd like _____ cheese, please.

Have you got _____ apple for me?

Here's _____ banana and _____ orange.

I'd like _____ peanut butter, please.

Would you like _____ baked beans on toast?

I'd like _____ egg and _____ toast for breakfast.

I'd like _____ roll and _____ juice, please.

6 *Fill in the words from the box.*

Martin: ___What's___ for breakfast?

Sally: _____ you like beans on toast?

Martin: Yuk! No, _____ you!

Sally: Well, what would you _____ then?

Martin: _____ some muesli or some cornflakes.

Sally: Sorry, we _____ got muesli or cornflakes.

Martin: No? _____ you got some yoghurt then?

Sally: Yes, I think so.

Martin: OK, I'd like some yoghurt and _____ apple.

Sally: Anything _____ ?

Martin: No, thank you. That's _____ .

fine
haven't
an
~~what's~~
I'd like
else
would
thank
like
have

7 *Put the sentences into the correct order.*

- [ ] OK. Toast and butter. Would you like some jam too?
- [ ] What would you like to drink?
- [ ] With milk?
- [1] Good morning, Mrs Martinez.
- [ ] Tea, please.
- [ ] Some toast and butter, please.
- [ ] Good morning, Sharon. What would you like for breakfast?
- [ ] No, thank you. Toast and butter is fine.
- [ ] Yes, please.

Toast and butter, please.

8 *Find the correct answers. Draw lines.*

Would you like some tea?	Yes, you can.
What would you like to eat for breakfast?	You can have muesli, yoghurt, toast or rolls.
Have you got some hot chocolate?	I'd like coffee, please.
What's for breakfast?	I'd like some cornflakes, please.
Can I make some baked beans on toast?	Yes, please.
What would you like to drink?	No, I'm sorry, we haven't.

Wordfield

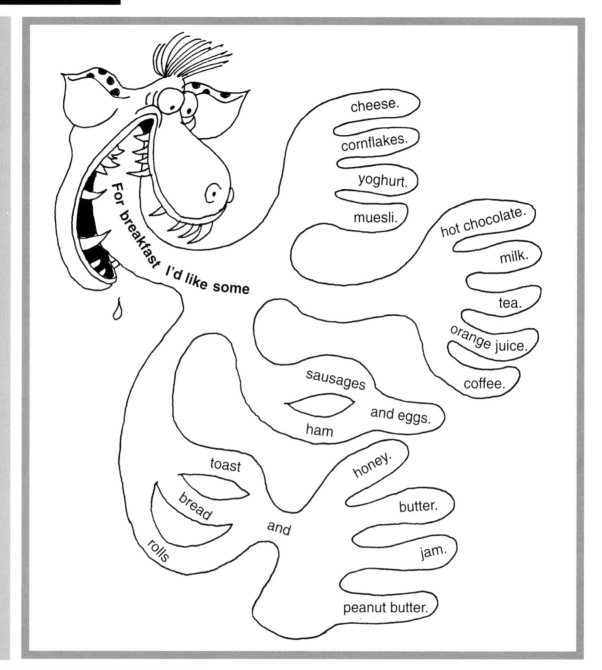

For breakfast I'd like some

cheese.

cornflakes.

yoghurt.

muesli.

hot chocolate.

milk.

tea.

orange juice.

coffee.

sausages and eggs.

ham

toast

honey.

butter.

bread

and

jam.

rolls

peanut butter.

Words in context

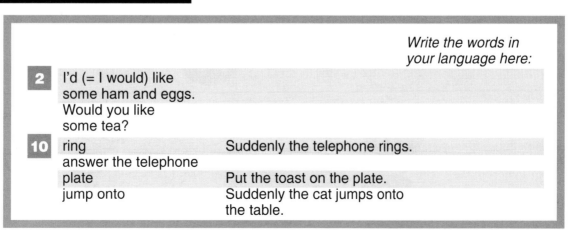

Write the words in your language here:

2 I'd (= I would) like some ham and eggs. Would you like some tea?

10 ring — Suddenly the telephone rings.

answer the telephone

plate — Put the toast on the plate.

jump onto — Suddenly the cat jumps onto the table.

UNIT 16

Brothers, sisters and friends

Revision

1 **Grammar**

Write the ordinal numbers.

19 <u>nineteenth</u>   23 _____   62 _____

8 _____   15 _____   100 _____

11 _____   59 _____   34 _____

6 _____   70 _____   81 _____

2 *Write down what the children like and what they don't like.*

Example:
Peter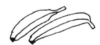

Peter likes apples, but he doesn't like bananas.

Peggy

Jonathan

Lisa

Kevin

Kylie

3 *Write down the dialogue.*

■

	Tina:	You and your cassettes. I want to watch the film.
	Stevie:	But I am here, and I can tell mum.
1	*Tina:*	Hey, Stevie. I want to watch TV. Stop that music.
	Stevie:	Tell me.
	Tina:	You are a real pest.
	Stevie:	The film on Sky Channel? Mum says it's not a film for you.
	Tina:	So tell her! You know what you are?
	Tina:	Mum says . . . mum says . . . She isn't here, is she?
	Stevie:	But I want to listen to my cassettes.

4 *Fill in:* **me – you – him – her – it – us – them**

■

Where is my bike? I can't see __it__ .

Where's Nora? I've got a book for _____ .

My best friend is Charles. I like _____ a lot.

Give me my cassettes. I want _____ back.

Our teacher is nice. She doesn't give _____ a lot of homework.

I can't do this exercise. Can you help _____ ?

Simon, here is some orange juice for _____ .

Where are Pam and Rick? I've got a letter for _____ .

Where's my schoolbag? I can't find _____ .

I've got a brother. Everybody calls _____ "Lolly".

me

you

him

her

it

us

you

them

5 *Fill in the blanks.*

■

I want to buy a book for __her__ (Wendy).

I want to buy a comic for _____ (Bob).

I eat _____ (baked beans) every day.

What can I give _____ (Sandra) to drink?

Mr Parker's cat wants _____ (the sausages) too.

I can't find _____ (Caroline).

I want to watch TV with _____ (Lester and Kate).

Can you help _____ (Clint)?

He looks at _____ (the boys) and smiles.

What is _____ (the word) in English?

6 *Write a text about Tim and Janet.*
Use the sentence starters from the grey boxes.

Tim: brother
name: Oliver
everybody: "Ollie"
age: 12
very nice
plays with him every day

Tim has got a brother.
His name is . . .
. . . calls him . . .
He is . . .
Tim thinks he . . .
He . . . every day.

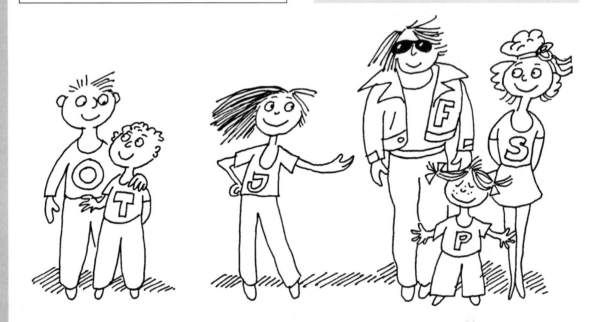

Janet: 1 brother, 2 sisters
names: Frank, Susan, Pamela
mum and dad: "Frankie", "Susie",
"Pam"
Frank: 18, Susan: 14, Pam: 5
Pam: mum's darling
Janet: Pam real pest
Janet: Frank great, gives her cassettes
Janet: Susan OK

Janet has got one brother and . . .
Their names are . . .
Their mum and dad call them . . .
Frank is eighteen, Susan . . .
. . .
Janet thinks Pam . . .
. . .
He . . .
Janet thinks . . .

7 **Pronunciation**

Word stress

One word in each list is different. Which is it?

■ ▢	■ ▢	■ ▢	■ ▢
funny	nothing	party	postman
alone	monster	problem	sweetie
shower	music	brother	around
homework	before	darling	window
honey	pencil	really	welcome
juicy	number	forget	boring
▢ ■	▢ ■	▢ ■	▢ ■

alone

Wordfield

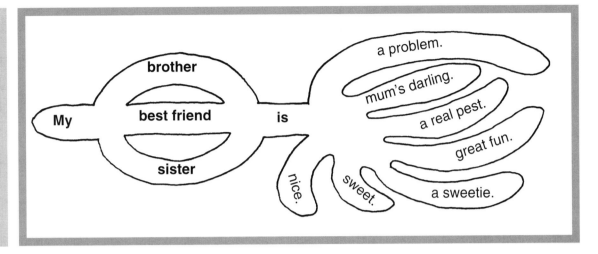

Words in context

Write the words in your language here:

1
name	My brother's name is Tom.
great	My sister is really great.
want to	He wants to sing.
rest	My brother wants to rest.

2
call	They call him Biker.
everybody	Everybody likes him.

6
front teeth	
is missing	A tooth is missing.
postman	
nobody	Nobody likes him.
be alone	She doesn't want to be alone.
maybe	Maybe you are right.
such a	He is such a pest

9
show	I want to see the show.
still	She is still up.
little one	
big one	
forget	Don't forget to write.
brush [brʌʃ]	Don't forget to brush your teeth.

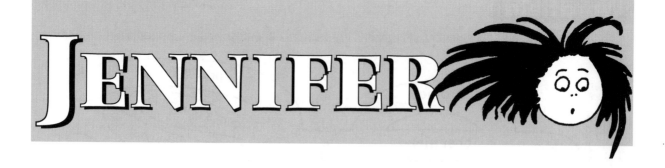

JENNIFER

Revision

1 **Grammar**

Write answers to the questions.

Do you walk to school? — **No, I don't.**

Can you play the piano? — No, I can't. ✓

Does your mother help you with your English homework? — Yes, she does. ✓

Can you speak Italian? — No, I can't. ✓

Have you got a brother? — Yes, I have ✓

Does your sister collect stamps? — No, I doesn't

Do your friends like English? — Yes, she do

Are you good at cooking? — Yes, I am ✓

Is your best friend good at skiing? — No, she is ✓

Do you like Jennifer's favourite story? — Yes, I Do ✓

2 **Grammar**

Fill in: **me – my – him – his – her – their**

Princess Cornelia has a friend. ___her___ name is Frederick. Cornelia loves ___him___, and he loves _____. She wants to marry _____, and he wants to marry _____. But _____ father, the king, says she must marry the sun, because he is the strongest. Cornelia says to the sun: " _____ father says I must marry the strongest." The sun answers: "The cloud is the strongest, because he can hide _____."

At the end of the story Cornelia and Frederick have a big party. All _____ friends come and everybody is happy.

3 Vocabulary

Can you find the opposites?
Write them down.

black	**white**	in	out ✓	big	small ✓
hot	clod cold ✓	sad	op Sad *happy*	woman	man ✓
boy	girl ✓	day	night	bad	happy good
ask	Answer	ugly	pritey ✓ *pretty*	hate	like ✓

4 *Put the sentences in the dialogues in the correct order.*

Dialogue 1: Jennifer and her mum

[8] M: Sorry, Jennifer, I cannot buy new jeans right now.

[3] J: Can I have a new pair of jeans?

[1] J: Mum, I have a problem.

[5] J: Because there are lots of stains on my jeans.

[2] M: What is it, Jennifer?

[7] J: But please, mum.

[4] M: A new pair of jeans? Why?

[6] M: No, Jennifer, I'm sorry.

Dialogue 2: Jennifer meets her friend Caroline

[5] C: I think they're super.

[2] J: I'm alright, thank you. And you?

[4] J: Do you like them?

[3] C: I'm OK. Are the jeans new?

[1] C: Hi, Jennifer. How are you doing?

Super!

5 *Draw lines.*

Why does Jennifer ask her mum for a new pair of jeans?	Because her mum cannot buy a new pair of jeans.
Why is Jennifer sad?	Because her friends think the birds on her jeans are great.
Why does Jennifer cut out the silk birds?	Because all the girls and boys have silk birds on their jeans.
Why is Jennifer happy?	Because there are stains on her jeans.
Why does Mrs Quentin smile?	Because she wants to sew them on her jeans.

75

6 *Can you find the sentences? Write them down.*

■ Example: **Jennifer wants a new pair of jeans.**

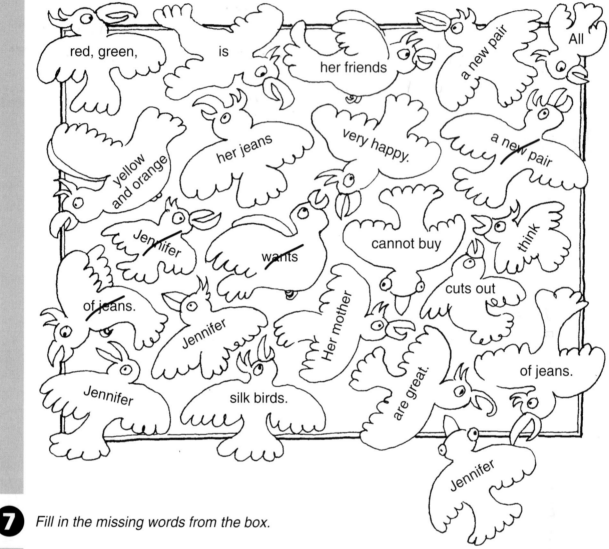

red, green,

is

her friends

a new pair

All

yellow and orange

her jeans

very happy.

a new pair

Jennifer

wants

cannot buy

think

of jeans.

Jennifer

Her mother

cuts out

of jeans.

Jennifer

silk birds.

are great.

Jennifer

7 *Fill in the missing words from the box.*

■ _____**Why doesn't**_____ Peter like the film? – Because he thinks the ending is not good.

Why can't I watch the film? – _____ you must help me in the kitchen.

Why _____ your brother so sad? – Because he can't go to the party.

Why can't you go to the shops for me? – Because I'm _____ my homework.

_____ is Linda not here? – Because she's in London with her mother.

Why can't you _____ the cassette? – Because I haven't got the money.

Why do you want a new blouse? – _____ my blouse has a grass stain on.

why
buy
is
because
doing
because
why
doesn't

76

8 **Pronunciation**

[s] or [z] ? Put these plurals into two lists.

apples books cabbages baskets cats desks examples dresses cornflakes
eyes films glasses paints socks jeans legs lots nights ideas nuggets

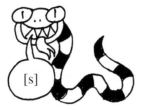

[s]   [z]

books _____ _____   apples _____ _____

_____ _____   _____ _____

_____ _____   _____ _____

_____ _____   _____ _____

Words in context

			Write the words in your language here:
2	stain		
	full of	Her jeans are full of stains.	
	unhappy	Jennifer is unhappy.	
	silk painting	Her class does silk painting.	
	cut out	She cuts the birds out.	
	sew on [səʊ]	She sews them on her jeans.	
	put on	Jennifer puts on her jeans with the birds.	
	a few days later		
5	why	Why do you like the story?	
	because	I like it because . . .	
	happy ending	There is a happy ending.	
	clever	Jennifer is very clever.	
8	princess		
	king		
	marry	The princess wants to marry Frederick.	
	must	You must marry the sun.	
	the strongest	Frederick is the strongest.	
	cloud		
	blow	The wind blows and blows.	
	bamboo		
	break	I cannot break the bamboo.	

What's on TV?

Revision

1

Grammar

Fill in the words from the box.

__Why__ can't I watch the film, dad? – Because it's time for bed.

_____ time is the news? – Half past seven.

_____'s the bracelet? – On the sofa.

_____ do you think quizzes are boring? – Because I can never answer the questions.

_____'s your birthday? – On April 24th.

_____ does the film start? – At five o'clock.

_____'s Jerry? – He's hiding behind the chair.

_____'s the time? – I don't know.

when
when
~~why~~
why
where
where
what
what

Where are my glasses?

2

Grammar

Fill in the words from the box.

at behind in ~~on~~ round in at away on in

Sharon is sitting __on__ the sofa _____ the living room watching her favourite TV programme "Kim's Island". Kim is an Indian boy. He lives _____ a tropical island. This week Kim is _____ the jungle. _____ a cave he finds a box. He opens it and finds two golden bracelets. Kim does not see the snake _____ him. Sharon sees the snake and shouts: "Kim! Kim!" Kim turns _____ and stands very still. He looks _____ the snake and the snake looks _____ him. Then the snake goes _____ . Kim is very happy. He gives Sharon one of the two golden bracelets.

3 **Grammar and vocabulary**

Fill in: **a – an – some**

Would you like _____ badges?

I've got _____ Italian flag.

I'd like _____ stamps, please.

Susan wants _____ new pair of jeans.

I'd like _____ orange T-shirt, please.

I've got _____ ink on my jacket.

Jennifer has got _____ oil stains on her jeans.

Would you like _____ milk?

Do you want _____ orange?

Can I have _____ peanut butter, please?

4 *Write the dialogues in the correct order.*

☐ Can I watch the film?

☐ Mum?

☐ I'm sorry. It's eight o'clock and time for bed.

☐ Yes, Peter?

☐ I think it's great.

☐ I don't like "Kim's Island". I think it's boring.

☐ "Kim's Island."

☐ What's your favourite programme?

5 *Write in the names of the programmes.*

1 _____ 5 _____

2 _____ 6 _____

3 _____ 7 _____

4 _____ 8 _____

6 *Write sentences. The numbers refer to the pictures in* 5 *.*

Tom /4/ boring: **Tom thinks romantic films are boring.**

Mary and Sandra /2/ great: _____

My father /7/ exciting: _____

I /3/ interesting: _____

John /1/ OK: _____

Sam and Janet /5/ exciting: _____

7 Look at this page from a TV magazine.
Fill in the names of the programmes from the box.

Newsweek   The girl and the rabbits   Sportsworld   In the jungle   The superquiz

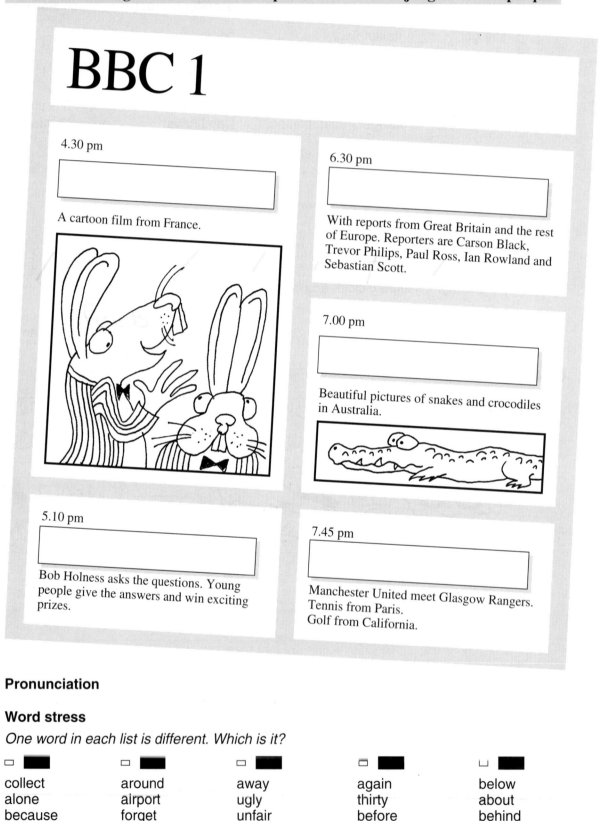

BBC 1

4.30 pm

A cartoon film from France.

6.30 pm

With reports from Great Britain and the rest of Europe. Reporters are Carson Black, Trevor Philips, Paul Ross, Ian Rowland and Sebastian Scott.

7.00 pm

Beautiful pictures of snakes and crocodiles in Australia.

5.10 pm

Bob Holness asks the questions. Young people give the answers and win exciting prizes.

7.45 pm

Manchester United meet Glasgow Rangers.
Tennis from Paris.
Golf from California.

8 Pronunciation

Word stress

One word in each list is different. Which is it?

☐ ■	☐ ■	☐ ■	☐ ■	☐ ■
collect	around	away	again	below
alone	airport	ugly	thirty	about
because	forget	unfair	before	behind
cabbage	guitar	July	cassette	bathroom
■ ☐	■ ☐	■ ☐	■ ☐	■ ☐

cabbage _____ _____ _____ _____

Wordfields

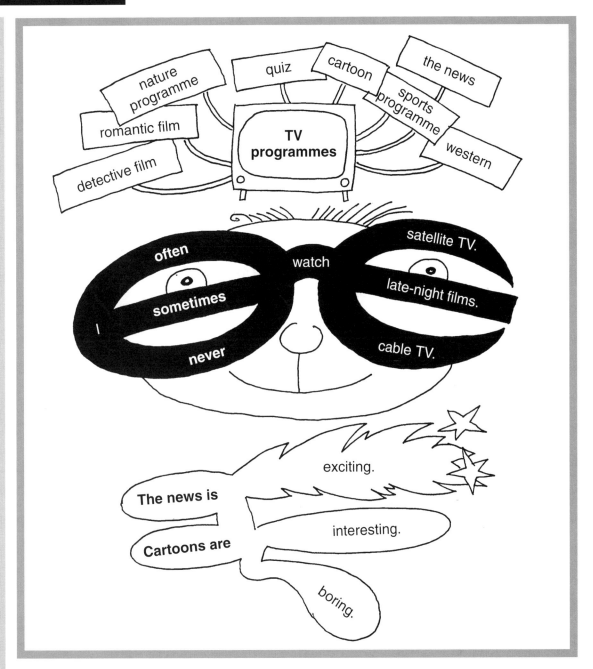

Words in context

5	young	Kim is a young Indian boy.
	live	
	tropical island	He lives on a tropical island.
	cave	Kim finds a cave in the jungle.
	golden bracelet	
	['breɪslɪt]	
6	cup of tea	Would you like a cup of tea?

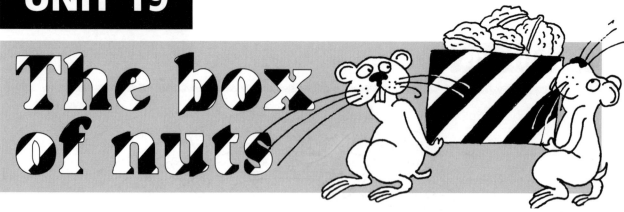

UNIT 19

The box of nuts

Revision

1 **Grammar**

Fill in the words from the box in the correct form.

| ~~feel~~ | ~~buy~~ | ~~look at~~ | ~~cut~~ | ~~do~~ | ~~sew~~ | ~~have~~ | smile |

Jennifer's mother can't ___**buy**___ new jeans.

Jennifer ___feels___ very unhappy because her jeans are full of stains.

Jennifer ___cuts___ out the silk birds.

Jennifer ___sews___ the silk birds on the jeans where the stains are.

Jennifer's friends ___look at___ her jeans.

On Sunday night Jennifer ___has___ a dream.

On Monday Jennifer's class ___does___ silk painting.

Mrs Quentin, Jennifer's teacher, ___smiles___ . ✓

2 **Grammar**

Fill in the words from the box.

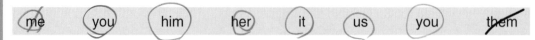

(~~me~~) (you) (him) (her) (it) (us) (you) ~~them~~

The Binhams are in the field. The dog is with **them**.

I think I can open the door. Give ___me___ the key.

Carol is happy because Steven makes baked beans on toast for ___her___.

Muesli for breakfast? I don't like ___it___ .

Where is George? Tell ___him___ to get up.

Give me an American stamp, Amy, and I'll give ___you___ a French stamp.

We can't do the exercise. Please help ___us___ .

Peter, Mary, come here! Mother wants to say hallo to ___you___.

3 **Vocabulary**

What words go together?

do   answer

put on   cook

have   brush

listen to   watch

the homework   my T-shirt

sausages   my cassettes   my teeth

TV

a cup of tea   the telephone

4 **Vocabulary**

Find the six breakfast words.

a a a a e e i j k l m n o s s s t t t u
a a c e f i k l l l m m m o r r s s

_____ _____

_____ _____

_____ _____

5 *Fill in the missing words.*

Crickwood is a small _p a l ec_ (place) in the west of England.

In the _woods_ and fields around Crickwood there are many _animals_.

There are also three _hamsters_. They like _nuts_ very much.

So they _steal_ some nuts from Mrs Binham. They take the nuts with them to a

pond. But Dave, one of the hamsters, is very _tired_ and he drops a

lot of nuts into the _grass_.

Pam and Mike _send_ Dave away and then they _eat_ all the nuts.

83

6 *Look at the pictures. Then match them with the speech bubbles.*

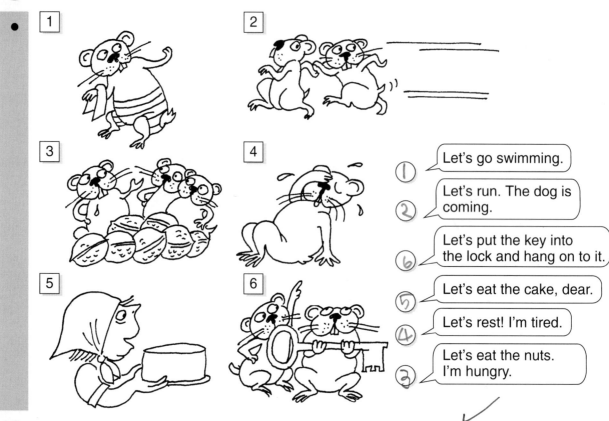

1
2
3
4
5
6

① Let's go swimming.

② Let's run. The dog is coming.

⑥ Let's put the key into the lock and hang on to it.

⑤ Let's eat the cake, dear.

④ Let's rest! I'm tired.

③ Let's eat the nuts. I'm hungry.

7 *Find the words.*

Joe Binham lives on a _farm_ near Crickwood.

The hamsters swim in the _pond_ .

There are lots of animals in the _woods_ .

Pam is a _hamster_ .

In the fields near Crickwood there also live _foxs_ .

Let's put the key into the _into the lock_ .

The hamsters all like _nuts_ .

8 *Look at the drawings and write down the words.*

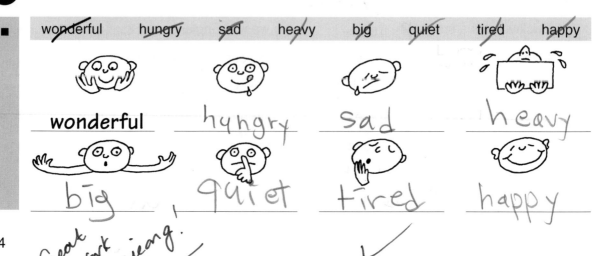

wonderful   hungry   sad   heavy   big   quiet   tired   happy

wonderful   hyngry   sad   heavy

big   quiet   tired   happy

Great work Hajeong!

84

9 **Pronunciation**

Sort out the words.

orange switch cabbage chair watch juggle ketchup June nature sausage much

[dʒ]		[tʃ]	
orange	_____	_____	_____
_____	_____	_____	_____
_____	_____	_____	_____

Wordfields

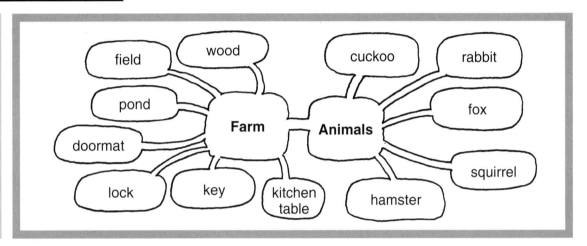

Words in context

*Write the words in
your language here:*

3

place	a small place
in the west	in the west of England
wife	Joe's wife helps him in the fields.
bake a cake	Every Saturday Mrs Binham bakes a chocolate cake.
if	
hang on to	The hamsters hang on to the key.
steal	The hamsters steal the nuts.
near	near the pond
heavy ['hevi]	The box is very heavy.
fall down	Dave is tired and falls down.

5

son	His son is eleven.
excited [ik'saɪtɪd]	Joe's son is very excited when the dog brings the hamster.
another	Let's read another story.
deep	The fox runs deep into the wood.
hear	Dave can hear a cuckoo.
bring	The squirrel brings Dave a lot of nuts.

6

| wait for | Wait for me, Dave! |
| look for | Let's look for nuts. |

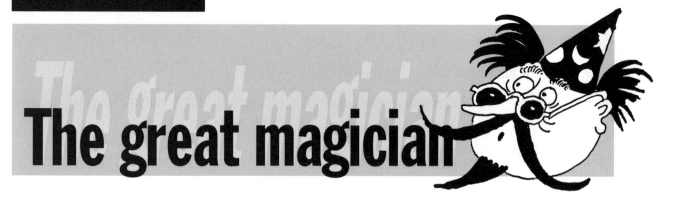

The great magician

Revision

1 **Grammar**

Write down the sentences in the correct order.

never/I/sports programme/watch/the
"Golden Mountains"/programme/My/is/favourite
think/news/boring/the/is/I
to/films/the jungle/tropical islands/about/I/and/like/watch
don't/watching/in/I/morning/like/TV/the
likes/Harry/on/not/are/many/westerns/but/TV/there

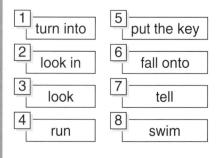

like / I /
books /
reading /
always

2 **Vocabulary**

Write in the correct numbers.

1	turn into	5	put the key
2	look in	6	fall onto
3	look	7	tell
4	run	8	swim

○	in the pond	②	home
○	into the lock	○	horrible
○	the grass	○	the telephone book
○	lots of stories	①	a fish

3 **Grammar and vocabulary**

Fill in the words from the box.

My __favourite__ TV programme is "Farm on the Hill".

I _____ watch sport programmes.

Kim gives Sharon a golden _____ .

Sharon sees the snake and _____ : "Kim! Kim!"

I _____ romantic films.

_____ you like some orange juice?

Kim _____ round and sees the snake.

In a _____ in the jungle he finds a golden box.

shouts

cave

~~favourite~~

hate

never

would

turns

bracelet

4 *Put the text into the correct order.*

☐ The magician, Frank Osbert, wants to help them.
☐ But now he can speak!
☐ The dog has pink ears and a yellow nose.
[1] The children are in the park with their dog, Blackie.
☐ Then he turns him into a dog again.
☐ They see that Blackie is drinking something horrible.
☐ Suddenly he shrinks.
☐ The children want to help Blackie, so they phone a magician.
☐ First he turns Blackie into a fish.

5 *Fill in:* **this – that**

Let's take _____ bottle here.
_____ is our teacher's new car over there.
Look here. In _____ book there is a picture of my sister.
The exercises on _____ page here are not very difficult.
Please bring me _____ red T-shirt over there.
_____ man near the tree is Peter's dad.

6 *Find the correct answers. Write the numbers against the answers on the right.*

[1] What's Blackie doing?
[2] Can we ask dad?
[3] How do we find a magician?
[4] Can I help you?
[5] Quick, get some water.
[6] Can you come at three o'clock?
[7] What's your telephone number?
[8] Do you want this bottle here?

☐ Let's look in the telephone book.
☐ Five-nine-seven-three-one-four.
☐ Yes, we have a problem with our dog.
☐ He is drinking something.
☐ No, that green bottle on the shelf.
☐ Here you are.
☐ No, let's ask mum.
☐ Yes, three o'clock is fine.

7 *Write down the telephone call in the correct order.*

☐ *Patrick:* Five-nine-seven-three-one-four.
☐ *Linda:* Well, erm, we've got a problem with our dog. Can we come and see you?
[1] *Patrick:* Ah, here is a magician. Let's phone him.
☐ *Osbert:* Yes, of course. Can you come right now?
☐ *Linda:* What's his phone number?
☐ *Linda:* Alright. I'll phone him. Five . . . nine . . . seven . . . three . . . one . . . four.
☐ *Linda:* Yes, we can.
☐ *Osbert:* Frank Osbert. Can I help you?

8 *Look at the pictures. Write down the story.*

★

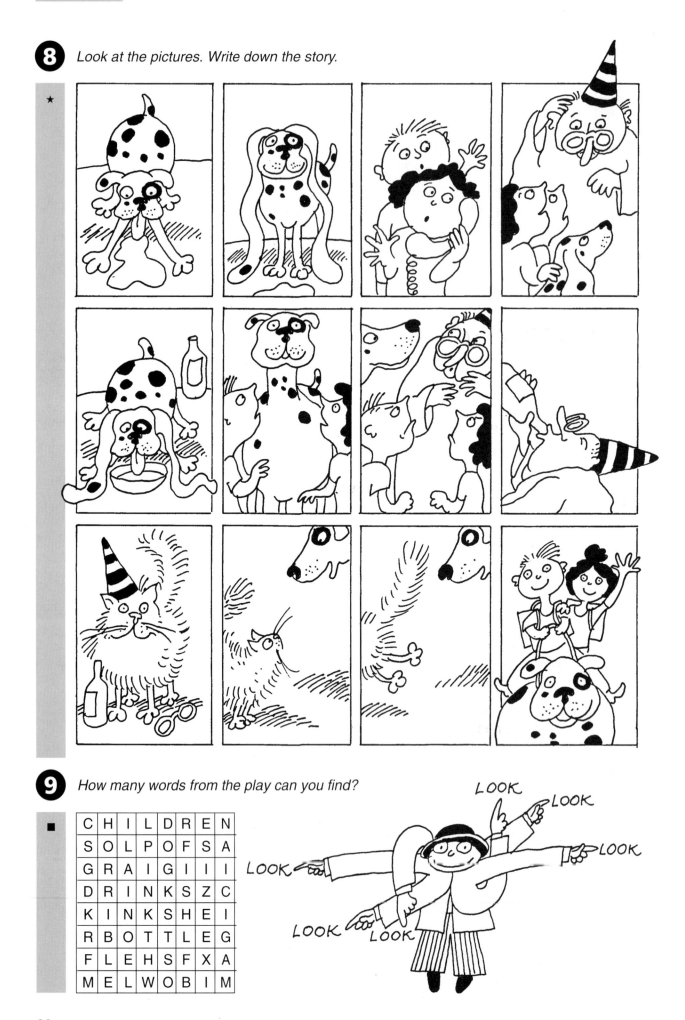

9 *How many words from the play can you find?*

■

C	H	I	L	D	R	E	N
S	O	L	P	O	F	S	A
G	R	A	I	G	I	I	I
D	R	I	N	K	S	Z	C
K	I	N	K	S	H	E	I
R	B	O	T	T	L	E	G
F	L	E	H	S	F	X	A
M	E	L	W	O	B	I	M

LOOK LOOK LOOK LOOK LOOK LOOK

10 Pronunciation

Odd man out

One word in each bottle is wrong. Underline it.

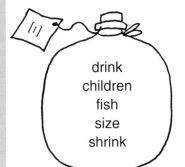

[ɪ]

drink
children
fish
size
shrink

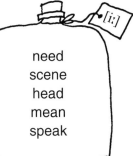

[iː]

need
scene
head
mean
speak

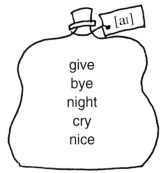

[aɪ]

give
bye
night
cry
nice

Words in context

*Write the words in
your language here:*

2

magician [məˈdʒɪʃən]	
children	
park	The children are in the park.
drink	Our dog never drinks milk.
horrible	The picture looks horrible.
shrink	Suddenly the dog starts shrinking.
size	What size are your jeans?
at home	The children are at home.
need	I need your help.
telephone book	
bottle	Give me the green bottle.
shelf	It's on the shelf.
Goodbye!	
happen	What is happening?
quick	
turn into	He's turning into a cat.
fish	
Oh dear!	
pour	Pour the water into the bowl.
Gosh!	
a little bit	
this	Do you want this bottle here?
that	No, that bottle on the shelf.

4

bat

UNIT 21
The elephant, the hippo and the mouse

Revision

1 **Grammar**

Fill in the correct words from the box.

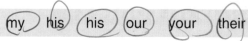

my   his   his   our   your   their

George, Willie and Fred like _their_ island very much. The elephant and the hippo are always happy. Every morning they say to Fred: "Bring us _our_ breakfast." Fred is not happy about _his_ job. "I don't want to make _your_ breakfast every day," he says to George and Willie. So one day he plays a trick on them. Now he says to George and Willie: "Bring me _my_ breakfast!" And every morning George and Willie must bring him _his_ breakfast. Clever Fred!

2 **Vocabulary**

Write down the words.

A is for **apple** .

B is for _Bat_ .

C is for _Cat_ .

D is for _Dog_ .

E is for _Egg_ .

F is for _Frog_ .

G is for _Gorilla_ .

H is for _Hippo_ .

I is for _insect_ .

J is for _Jogging_ .

K is for _Kate_ .

L is for _lemon_ .

M is for _Mom_ .

N is for _No_ .

O is for _octopus_ .

P is for _pan_ .

Q is for _Queen_ .

R is for _Rabbit_ .

S is for _swim_ .

T is for _Tim_ .

U is for _Use_ .

V is for _video_ .

W is for _water_ .

X is for **Xmas (= Christmas)**

Y is for _You_ .

Z is for **ZOO** .

90

3 **Word ladders**

★

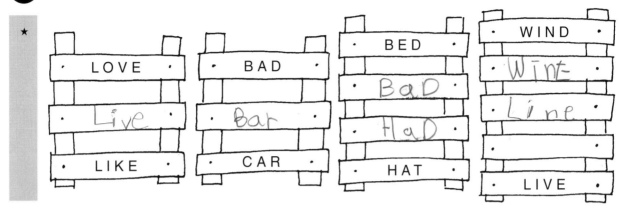

LOVE
Live
LIKE

BAD
Bar
CAR

BED
BaD
HaD
HAT

WIND
WinT
Line
LIVE

4 *Can you find the animals? Go along the lines.*

★

Example: **horse**, Dog, Frog, snake paRRot

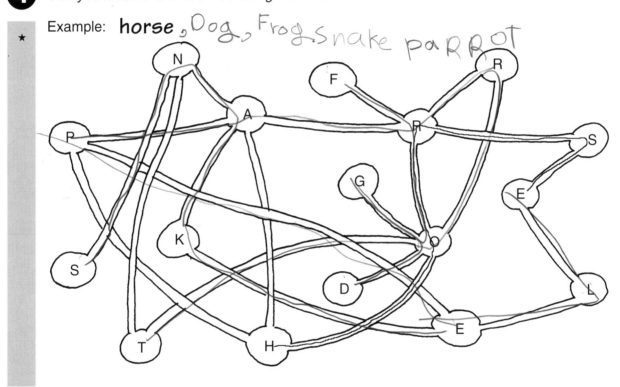

5 *Write sentences about the story.*

★

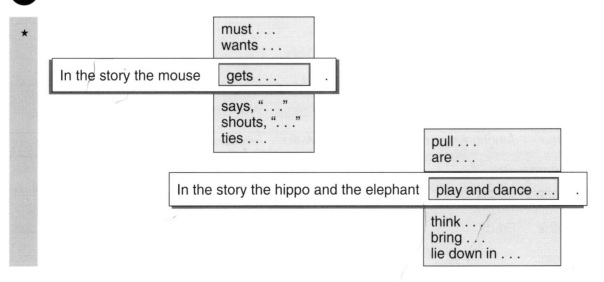

must . . .
wants . . .

In the story the mouse gets . . . .

says, " . . ."
shouts, " . . ."
ties . . .

pull . . .
are . . .

In the story the hippo and the elephant play and dance . . . .

think . . .
bring . . .
lie down in . . .

6 *Write down the sentences.*

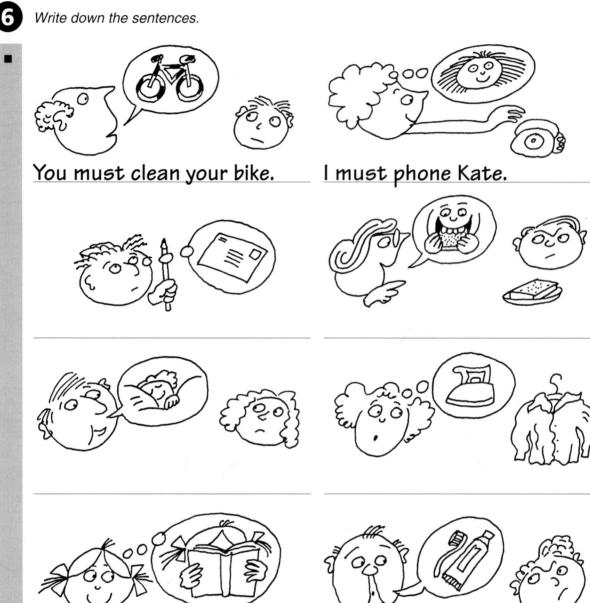

You must clean your bike.   I must phone Kate.

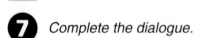

7 *Complete the dialogue.*

George: Fred, I'm hungry.

Fred: Alright. _____?

George: I want eight bananas.

Fred: Alright. Anything to drink?

George: Yes. _____.

Fred: Alright.

Willie: Fred, _____.

Fred: _____?

Willie: _____ and

        _____ bottles of juice.

Fred: Why do you want so much food?

Willie: Because I _____.

Fred: _____ stronger.

Willie: Haha! I am _____.

Fred: Let's see. Let's _____ rope.

Willie: OK.

8 Pronunciation

Write the words in three lists.

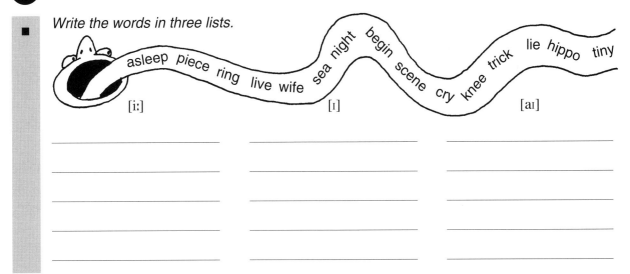

asleep piece ring live wife sea night begin scene cry knee trick lie hippo tiny

[iː]   [ɪ]   [aɪ]

_____   _____   _____

_____   _____   _____

_____   _____   _____

_____   _____   _____

Words in context

		Write the words in your language here:
3 hippo		
sea		
far across	The island is far across the sea.	
sand	They dance in the sand.	
make the bed		
strong	The elephant is strong.	
make a plan	One night Fred makes a plan.	
play a trick	Fred plays a trick on George and Willie.	
early	Fred gets up early in the morning.	
long		
rope	Let's pull the rope.	
soon		
stronger than	Is Fred stronger than George?	
begin	The elephant begins to laugh.	
tiny ['taɪni]	Fred is a tiny mouse.	
tie around	Fred ties the rope around George's leg.	
top	Fred runs to the top of the hill.	
lie down	The elephant and the hippo lie down.	
fall asleep		
wake up	The elephant wakes up next morning.	
to himself	He says it to himself.	
from that time on		
friendly	George and Willie are very friendly now.	
piece	They bring him a little piece of cheese.	

UNIT 22

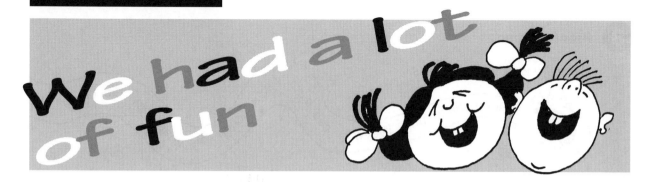

Revision

1 Grammar

Fill in: **why – how – what – where – when**

<u>How</u> can we get into the house? – I've got a key.

_____ is his birthday party? – On Saturday at five.

_____ are my jeans? – I think they are under your bed.

_____ don't you like the story? – Because there is no happy ending.

_____ does your school start? – At nine.

_____ 's your sister's name? – Jennifer.

_____ is your sister? – Oh, she's fine.

_____ does Joe live? – He lives in Crickwood.

_____ does Fred eat for breakfast? – An apple and a little piece of cheese.

_____ does Jennifer look so happy? – Because all her friends like her new jeans.

2 Vocabulary

When are their birthdays? Write down sentences.

Example: **Tom's birthday is on January 31ˢᵗ.**

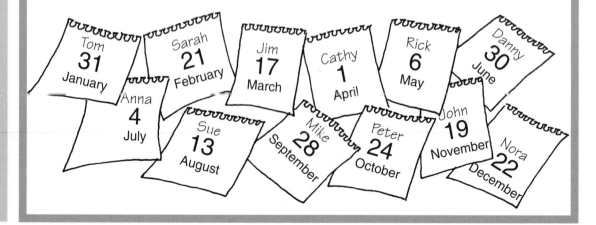

3 *Fill in the missing forms.*

have	**had**		gave	see	
listened		I am	I	go	
they are	they		played		said
take		jump		she is	she

4 *Fill in the words (past forms).*

Yesterday I h_ _ a dream. In my dream I s_ _ Peregrine,

the penguin.

He t_ _ _ me to a swimming pool, and there w_ _ a

group of penguins. They p_ _ _ _ _ really great rock and

roll music. Then Peregrine t_ _ _ me by the hand and we

j_ _ _ _ _ into the pool. Then we h_ _ something to

drink and l_ _ _ _ _ _ _ to the band. It w_ _ great!

Suddenly my mum s_ _ _ : "Time for school!"

So I w_ _ _ to school.

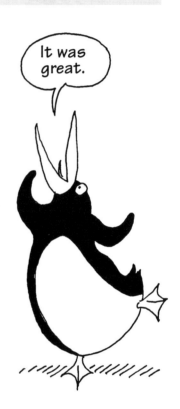

It was
great.

5 *Fill in the words from the box.*

Sandra's 12th birthday __was__ on the 31st of May. At her party there

_____ Susan, Kelly and me.

We _____ hot dogs and juice. Sandra _____ a big birthday cake.

There _____ twelve candles on it.

Sandra's mother _____ her a lovely red sweater.

Her father _____ her a ring.

I _____ her a book.

First we _____ some cake.

Then we _____ to Sandra's room.

We _____ to cassettes and _____ a lot of fun.

| ~~was~~ had |
| had had |
| had gave |
| gave gave |
| were were |
| listened |
| went |

6 *Look at the pictures. Write the story.*

★

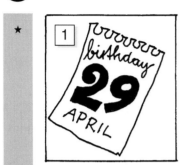 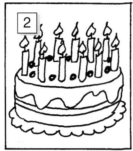 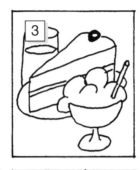 

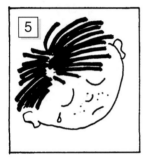 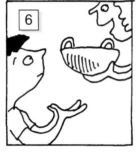 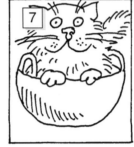 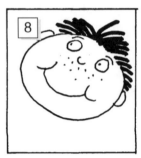

7 *Find the words.*

The penguins play in a . . .

In this book there are many . . .

Jimmy likes . . . music.

Past form of "take"

Past form of "have"

Past form of "say"

Past form of "give"

I went to a party . . .

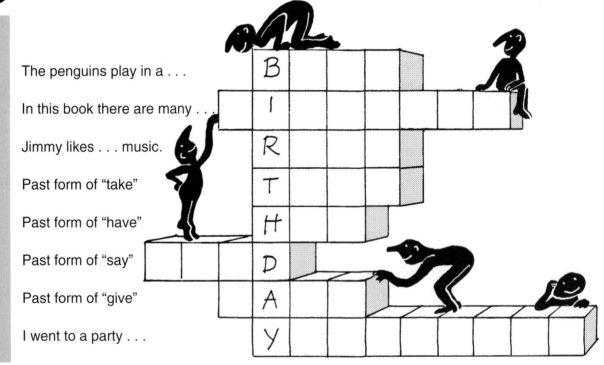

8 **Pronunciation**

[w]: Underline the odd ones out.

work	write	Wednesday	with
wrist	wind	where	were
week	word	wrong	would
woman	wear	what	wrap

Wordfield

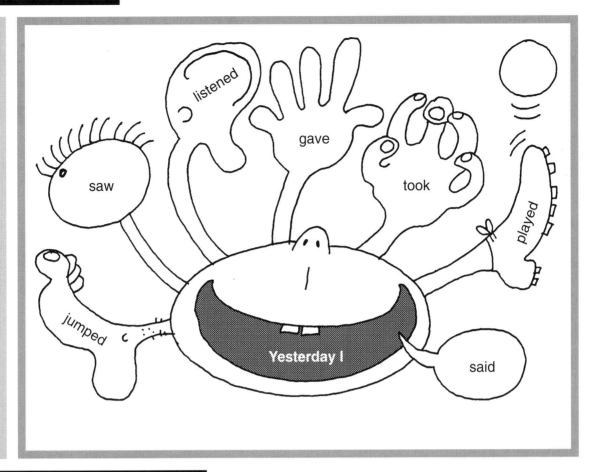

Words in context

Write the words in your language here:

1

were	There were penguins at the swimming pool.
was	It was on a Thursday.
went	We went to the swimming pool.
had	We had a lot of fun.

2

yesterday	Yesterday I had a dream.
band	The penguins played in a band.
cool	The band was really cool.

Take me by the hand.

3

took a photo

4

different from	This picture is different from what Martin said.
fish fingers	

UNIT 23

The pink racket

Revision

1 Grammar

Fill in the words from the box.

| me | him | her | her | it | us | them | them |

This racket is for Helen. Give _____ to _____ .

John has got a problem with his racket. Can you help _____?

On Helen's birthday her dad gave _____ a big box.

Here are two boxes for Helen. Please give _____ to her, but do not open _____ .

Our coach is very friendly. He is always very nice to _____.

I don't like playing tennis. Please don't ask _____ to play with you.

2 Vocabulary

Fill in the missing words.

Helen: Hi, Sheila.

Sheila: Hi, Helen. How _____ your birthday?

Helen: It _____ OK, _____ dad _____ me a _____ I didn't like.

Sheila: _____ was it?

Helen: A tennis racket.

Sheila: _____ don't you like it?

Helen: _____ I hate playing tennis.

3 Vocabulary

Find the words that go together and write down sentences.

Example: **Fred played a trick on Willie and George.**

fall	a trick	feel	jeans
bake	into a mouse	watch	sausages
open	asleep	listen to	unhappy
turn	a cake	put on	TV
play	the door	cook	cassettes

98

4 *Read through Helen's story and fill in the words in their past forms.*

When I was a schoolgirl, my family l_ _ _ _ tennis. They w_ _ _ very good players, and they p_ _ _ _ _ every weekend. I w_ _ _ _ _ _ _ them every weekend, but I d_ _ not like it. I l_ _ _ _ reading and watching TV. On my birthday, dad g_ _ _ me a tennis racket. So we w_ _ _ to play together, but I h_ _ _ _ it. That evening I w_ _ _ to my room and l_ _ _ _ _ _ at my racket. Then I p_ _ the racket into a box, and g_ _ _ it back to dad. When he f_ _ _ _ the box, he d_ _ not say a word. And after that, when my family w_ _ _ playing tennis, I s_ _ at home and r_ _ _ _ my books and w_ _ _ _ _ _ _ TV.

5 *How many sentences can you make? Write them down.*

Example: **Helen didn't like playing tennis.**

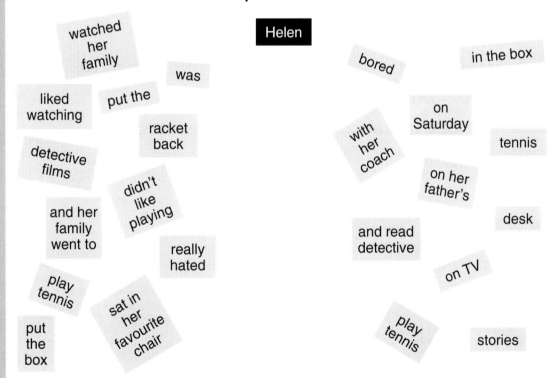

6 *Can you find the ten irregular past forms?*

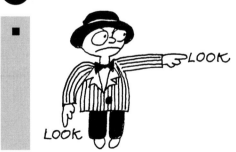

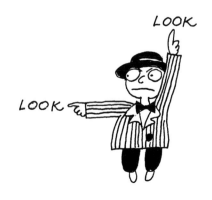

LOOK

T	W	E	N	T	E	N
K	A	H	P	U	T	W
O	S	A	I	D	S	E
O	A	D	D	A	E	R
T	T	G	A	V	E	E

7 *Write down the words from the story "The pink racket".*

acrtke _____   hccao   _____

lepary _____   dbreo   _____

mssah _____   ndeeekw _____

8 **Pronunciation**

Write the words in three lists.

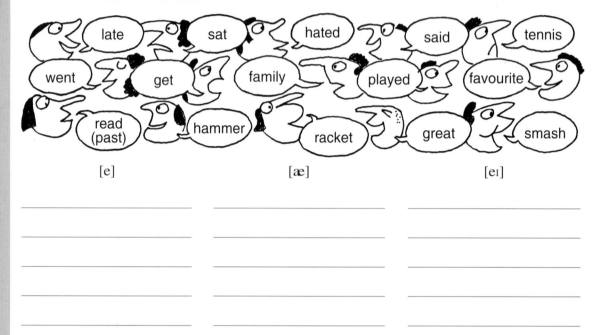

late   sat   hated   said   tennis

went   get   family   played   favourite

read (past)   hammer   racket   great   smash

[e]   [æ]   [eɪ]

_____   _____   _____

_____   _____   _____

_____   _____   _____

_____   _____   _____

_____   _____   _____

Words in context

Write the words in your language here:

2		
player	She was a good player.	
weekend	They play tennis at weekends.	
come along	"Come along," they said.	
bored	Helen was bored.	
detective story	She liked reading detective stories.	
tennis racket		
coach		
together	They played tennis together	
evening	In the evening John often watches TV.	
stupid	What a stupid present!	
smash	I'd like to smash the racket.	
to herself	"I'd like to smash it," she said to herself.	
no longer		

Greedy Oliver

Revision

1

Grammar

Fill in the missing words.

_____ do you want? – An apple, please.

_____ much are the jeans? – £25.

_____ is my sweater? – Under the chair.

_____ flavour is it? – Strawberry.

_____ is the noise coming from? – From the kitchen.

_____ is your birthday? – On the 25th of March.

_____ is making that noise? – Cathy is playing her guitar.

_____ is the time? – It's five past seven.

_____ many stickers have you got? – About seventy.

2

Grammar

How many questions can you make?

Example: **Do monkeys like apples?**

Is	they	collect	at three o'clock?
Do	she	come	stamps?
Are	you	want	me?
Can	monkeys	help	apples?
Does		good at	an apple?
		like	swimming?
		swim?	some ketchup?
		alright?	milk?
		often	at our school?
		new	stamps?
			watch nature programmes?

3 *Fill in the missing forms of the verbs.*

have | had ✓ | | tood | take took | | dav give | gave
think thought | thinked | see | saw ✓ | | go | geos ment
saided say | said | do | does did | | get ✓ | got
sated sit | sat | find | found finded | | read | readed read
put | pad put | eat | ate ✓ | | buy | bought
fall | falled fell | | hided hid | | run | ran ✓

4 *Fill in the missing words from the box.*

fell   bought   took   saw   ate   ran over   gave   tried   went

Sally __took__ ✓ her grandma's dog for a walk. Grandma __gave__ her 50p.

Sally __went__ for a walk in the park. She __saw__ ✓ an ice-cream man.

Sally __ran over__ ✓ to the ice-cream man. She __bought__ ✓ an ice-cream cornet.

A big boy __tried__ ✓ to grab her cornet. The ice cream __fell__ ✓ onto

the grass. A dog __ate__ ✓ it.

5 *Fill in the missing words.*

Grandmother: Here you __are__ ✓ , Oliver.

Oliver: __thank__ ✓ you, grandma.

At the shop

Oliver: A cornet, __pleases__ ✓.

Shopkeeper: What flavour do you __got__ want ?

Oliver: Chocolate and vanilla.

Shopkeeper: __that's__ ✓ 50p.

Oliver: _____ you are.

Shopkeeper: Thank you.

Oliver: _____ .

Shopkeeper: Bye.

6 *Find the fourteen words that do not belong to the story. Write down the correct words.*

Oliver hated sweets. One day Oliver's grandmother gave me a cat. Oliver quickly ran over to the swimming pool. There he grabbed a bar of chocolate. He dropped the chocolate in the park. Then he went to Mrs Spencer's house and took her dog for a walk. Mrs Spencer bought Oliver a bike. So Oliver bought a tired bag of toffees. He ate the toffees in the shop. Then Oliver saw a monster eating a freezer. And Oliver saw ice-cream flowers dancing before his eyes. He ran over to the sweet shop and hid behind the cupboard.

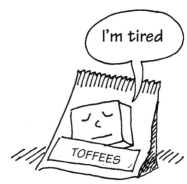
I'm tired
TOFFEES

hated → loved

_____ _____

_____ _____

_____ _____

_____ _____

_____ _____

7 *Look at the pictures and write down sentences about Cathy.*

Start like this: **Yesterday was Cathy's birthday.**

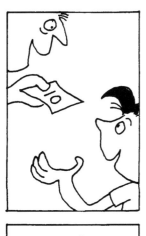 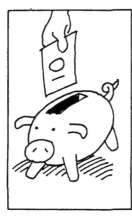 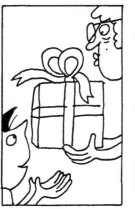 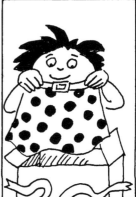

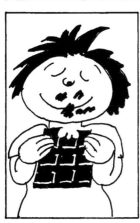 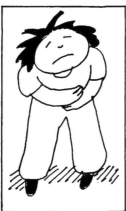 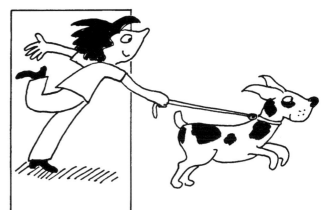

8 *Write down the correct sentences.*

- went to/her dog/house/Oliver/took/Mrs Spencer's/and/for a walk
to the sweet shop/hid/Oliver/the freezer/and/ran over/behind
the shopkeeper/Oliver/When/her back/opened/turned/the freezer
to grab/ice-cream cornets/Oliver/six/fell in/tried/and
helped/waited/she/out/Oliver/The shopkeeper/and then/for a minute
gave/50p/put it/The next time/he/Oliver/grandma/in his piggybank

9 **Pronunciation**

- *Sort out the words.*

thirty	there	think	through	them	Thursday	thief	they	thing	mother

[ð]	[θ]
_____	_____
_____	_____
_____	_____
_____	_____
_____	_____

Words in context

			Write the words in your language here:
2	bought	He bought an ice-cream cornet.	
	ran	She ran over to the shop.	
	ate	A dog ate the ice-cream cornet.	
	tried	She tried to open the door.	
	grab	He tried to grab the cornet.	
	went for a walk	John went for a walk in the park.	
	fell	The book fell on the floor.	
3	greedy	He was very greedy.	
	quickly	He quickly ran over to the shop.	
	thought	He thought, "I'd like some toffees."	
	hid	He hid behind the freezer.	
	freezing cold		

What are you going to do?

Revision

1

★

Grammar

How many questions can you make? Write them down.

Example: **What are you going to collect?**

| How
Where
What
Who
When | is
do you
many
are you
was
much | badges
stamps
going to
are
making | my scissors?
think?
collect?
stay with us?
want?
John?
your birthday?
do?
English book?
have you got?
the jeans?
that noise?
the time? |

2

■

Grammar

Find the sentences that go together. Write in the correct numbers.

1	What colour is your new mountain bike?	○ No, I don't.
2	Give me the red bottle.	○ 80p.
3	I like wearing trainers to school.	○ Yes, I'm fine, thanks.
4	What flavour is it?	○ So do I.
5	Are you alright?	○ Peppermint.
6	How much are the envelopes?	○ Here you are.
7	The red T-shirt is £12.	○ Yes, I think so.
8	Do parrots eat caterpillars?	① Stickers.
9	Is this Sue's bike?	○ Green.
10	Can you ride a horse?	○ Yes, she does.
11	What do you collect?	○ Karen is playing the guitar.
12	Does she like strawberry shake?	○ No, I can't.
13	Do you like coffee?	○ No, they don't.
14	Who is making that noise?	○ OK. I'll take it.

3 | **Grammar**

"s" or no "s"?

He **likes** _____ bananas. (like)

The elephant and the hippo _____ a plan. (make)

My brother doesn't _____ chicken. (eat)

The crocodile _____ a long list. (write)

Tom and Susan _____ home at half past five. (get)

My knee _____ . (hurt)

She _____ up at seven o'clock. (get)

They often _____ TV in the evening. (watch)

Does she _____ some coffee? (want)

With £5 she can _____ a lot of sweets. (buy)

He doesn't _____ his father's present. (like)

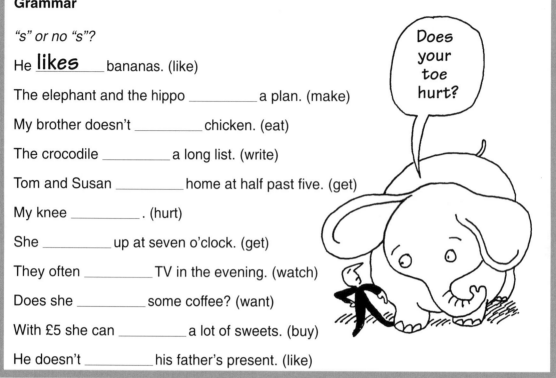

Does your toe hurt?

4 | *Fill in:* **am – are – is**

Sally _____ going to play tennis with Steven this afternoon.

Dad _____ going to take me to the circus on Sunday.

They _____ going to play cards with their grandmother on Saturday.

_____ you going to visit your friends in Scotland this weekend?

Where _____ he going to stay in London?

I _____ going to swap stamps with Liza this afternoon.

We _____ going to have a party next Saturday.

_____ they going to play volleyball this afternoon?

_____ he going to watch the film at half past six?

5 | *Find the words that go together and write down sentences.*

Example: **Let's do our homework now.**

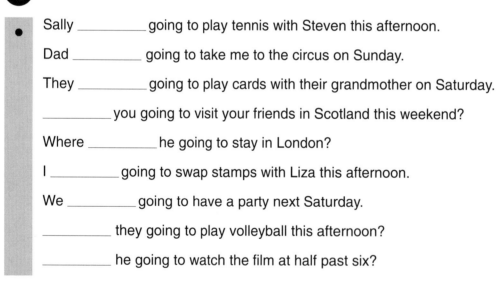

copy	a hamburger
climb	stamps
jump into	the sentences
do	off your face
clean	quiet!
wipe the ketchup	your knees
be	trees
order	the board
bend	the water
collect	our homework

6 *Write down what the children are going to do at the weekend.*

Example: **Jenny is going to take her dog for a walk.**

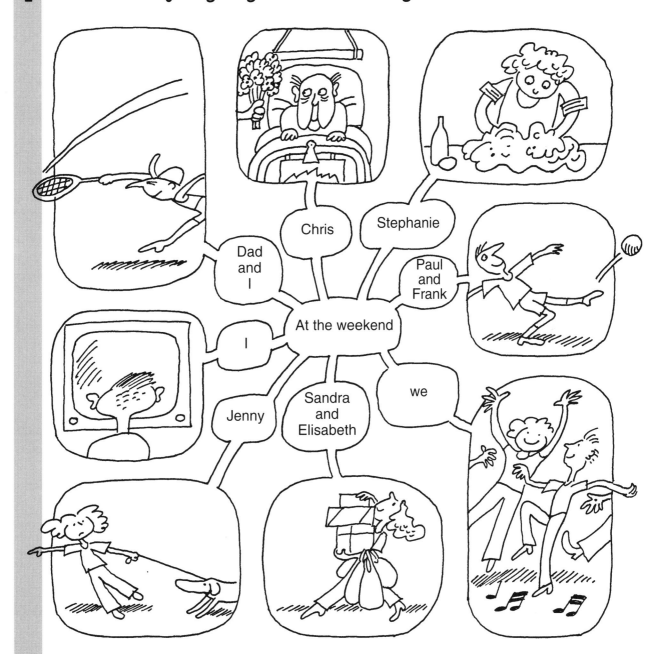

7 *Put the sentences in the correct order.*

▢ OK. Goodbye. See you at school

▢ Jennifer, I'm going to play table tennis with Penny this afternoon.
Would you like to come?

[1] Hallo, Jennifer.

▢ Bye.

▢ No, I'm sorry. I'm going to do the shopping with mum.

▢ Oh hi, Philip.

8 *There are seven groups of four words that rhyme. Look at the box and write the words down.*

bad	bread	cake	four	sew	me	more	head	bake	sad	tea	ache
		blow	said	had	door	see	take	show			

Group 1: cake, **bake, ache, take**

Group 2: dad, _____

Group 3: key, _____

Group 4: know, _____

Group 5: floor, _____

Group 6: red, _____

> My name rhymes with these things.

Words in context

Write the words in your language here:

2

afternoon	Let's play table tennis in the afternoon.	
wash	I'm going to wash our car in the afternoon.	
do the shopping		
grandfather		
hospital	Grandfather is in hospital.	
stay	We are going to stay in a hotel in London.	
visit	Let's visit John in hospital.	
Scotland		
play cards	We played cards yesterday.	
cinema	Jim took us to the cinema.	
Cup Final		
cheers	You can say "Bye" or "Cheers".	
Lucky you.		
lunch		
What a pity.		

3

model plane	We are going to make a model plane at the weekend.	
table tennis		
shopping centre		
Bye.		

5

ghost	There was a ghost in my room.	
let out	Don't let the dogs out.	
feed	I'm going to feed the parrots.	
bookworm ['bʊkwɜːm]		
knife [naɪf]	Don't touch the knife.	

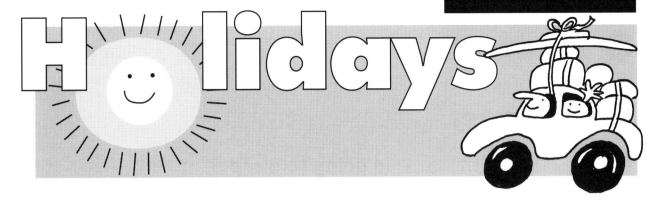

Holidays

Revision

1

★

Grammar

Fill in the past forms of the words in the box.

In the summer of 1993 I _____ in the USA with my mum

and my dad. First we _____ to New York. We

_____ there for a week. We_____ up the Statue

of Liberty, the Empire State Building and the World Trade Center.

We often _____ in Central Park and we _____ a lot

of shopping. My father _____ lots of books and I

_____ jeans and T-shirts and nice green shoes.

Then we _____ to Los Angeles. There we _____

Hollywood and Disneyland. We _____ a lot of fun. In

August we _____ a lot of places in California. After that

we _____ in San Francisco for a week.

My holidays in America _____ super.

I really want to go there again.

visit
visit
be
be
do
go
go
go
buy
buy
stay
stay
walk
have

Note
The Empire State Building has
102 storeys and is one of the
tallest buildings in New York.
World Trade Center: two gigantic
office buildings in New York.
Central Park: a park in the centre
of Manhattan.

2

★

Grammar

*Write a short text about what Helen did in
her last holidays.
Use words from the box.*

two weeks in a house in Italy	swimming	play tennis with her brother
eat a lot of ice cream	visit nice places	meet nice people
weekend at home	sleep late	read two books

3 Write sentences. What are they going to do in their summer holidays?
Use the verbs in the box.

| watch | play | visit | swim | stay at | ride | go | sleep |

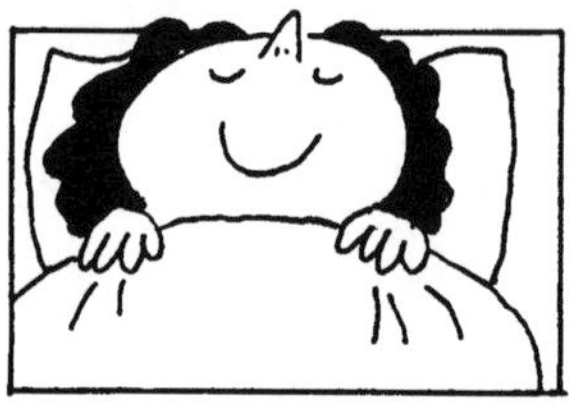

Susan **is going to sleep** _____

_____ a lot.

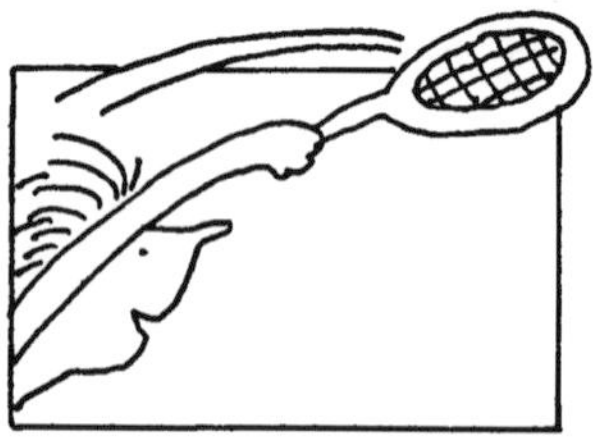

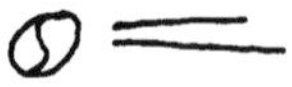

Cathy and Lisa _____

_____ a lot.

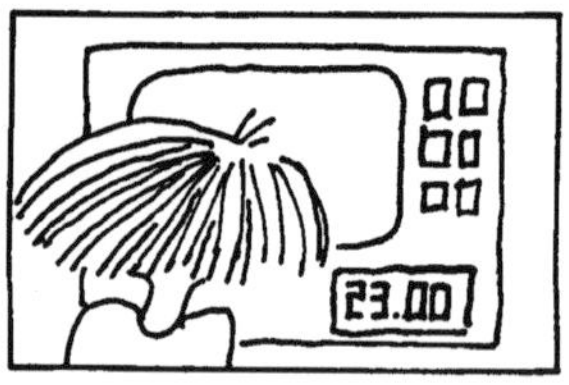

Nora _____

_____ a lot.

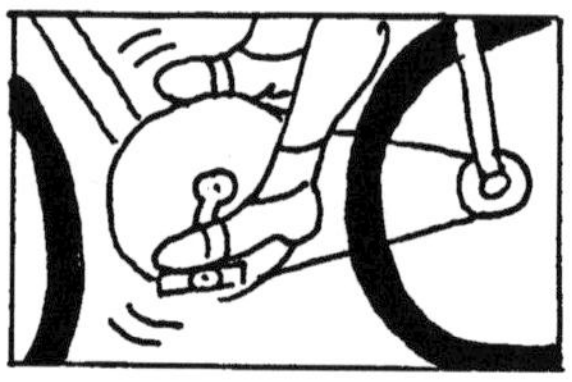

Kylie and her dad _____

_____ their bikes.

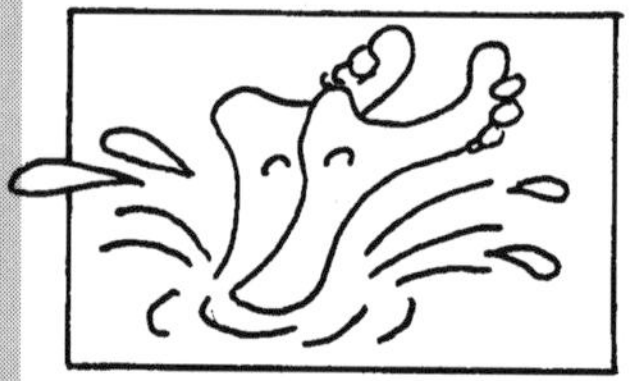

Jane and Fahim _____

_____ a lot.

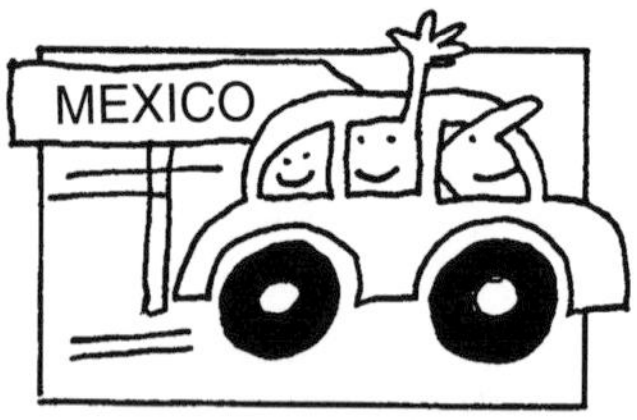

Sarah and her family _____

_____ .

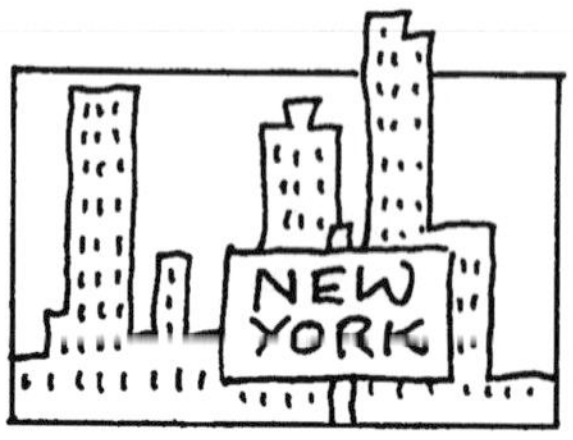

Our English teacher _____

_____ .

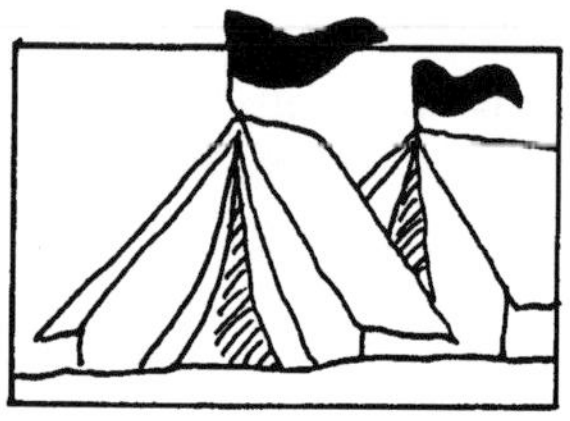

Maria, José and Anna _____

_____ .

4 *Who is going to do what? Write sentences.*

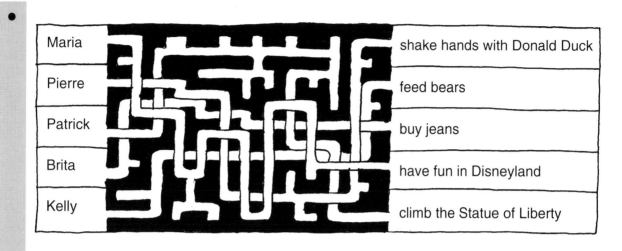

Maria	shake hands with Donald Duck
Pierre	feed bears
Patrick	buy jeans
Brita	have fun in Disneyland
Kelly	climb the Statue of Liberty

5 *Do you know the flags? Write down the words. Colour the flags.*

HANISPS

_____

GRATINNAIEN

_____

REGEK

_____

SHIRI

_____

SAULARTAIN

_____

NCAXIME

_____

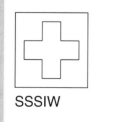

SSSIW

_____

Wordfield

Countries

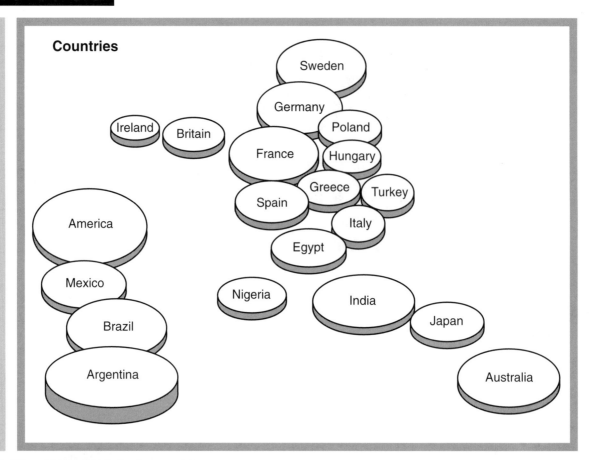

Sweden
Germany
Ireland
Britain
Poland
France
Hungary
Greece
Spain
Turkey
Italy
America
Egypt
Mexico
Nigeria
India
Japan
Brazil
Argentina
Australia

Words in context

Write the words in your language here:

3	flag	The Spanish flag is red, yellow and red.
4	in the middle	Our flag is white in the middle.
	cross	There's a cross on the Swiss flag.
	difficult	
5	holiday	A holiday in the USA is great.
	Statue of Liberty ['stætʃuːvlɪbəti]	
	zoo	I'm going to see the bears in San Diego zoo.
6	spend	I'm going to spend my holidays at home.
	bike tour	I'm going to go on a bike tour with dad.
	sleep late	
	stay up late	